THE TOP 100 DRUGS

KU-224-550

CLINICAL PHARMACOLOGY AND PRACTICAL PRESCRIBING

Andrew Hitchings BSc(Hons) MBBS MRCP FHEA
Clinical Research Fellow
St George's, University of London
Specialty Registrar (ST7) in Clinical Pharmacology,
General Medicine and Intensive Care Medicine
St George's Healthcare NHS Trust, London, UK

Dagan Lonsdale BSc(Hons) MBBS MRCP FHEA
Academic Clinical Fellow
St George's, University of London
Specialty Registrar (ST3) in Clinical Pharmacology,
General Medicine and Intensive Care Medicine
St George's Healthcare NHS Trust, London, UK

Daniel Burrage BSc(Hons) MBBS MRCP FHEA
Academic Clinical Fellow
St George's, University of London
Specialty Registrar (ST3) in Clinical Pharmacology and General Medicine
St George's Healthcare NHS Trust, London, UK

Emma Baker PhD FRCP
Professor of Clinical Pharmacology
St George's, University of London
Consultant Physician
St George's Healthcare NHS Trust, London, UK

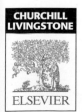

CHURCHILL
LIVINGSTONE

ELSEVIER

Edinburgh   London   New York   Oxford   Philadelphia   St. Louis   Sydney   Toronto   2015

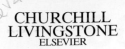

CHURCHILL LIVINGSTONE
ELSEVIER

© 2015 Elsevier Ltd. All rights reserved.

ISBN   978-0-7020-5516-4
  Reprinted 2015
eBook ISBN   978-0-7020-5515-7

British Library Cataloguing in Publication Data
A catalogue record for this book is available from the British Library

Library of Congress Cataloging in Publication Data
A catalog record for this book is available from the Library of Congress

Notices

Knowledge and best practice in this field are constantly changing. As new research and experience broaden our understanding, changes in research methods, professional practices, or medical treatment may become necessary.

Practitioners and researchers must always rely on their own experience and knowledge in evaluating and using any information, methods, compounds, or experiments described herein. In using such information or methods they should be mindful of their own safety and the safety of others, including parties for whom they have a professional responsibility.

With respect to any drug or pharmaceutical products identified, readers are advised to check the most current information provided (i) on procedures featured or (ii) by the manufacturer of each product to be administered, to verify the recommended dose or formula, the method and duration of administration, and contraindications. It is the responsibility of practitioners, relying on their own experience and knowledge of their patients, to make diagnoses, to determine dosages and the best treatment for each individual patient, and to take all appropriate safety precautions.

To the fullest extent of the law, neither the Publisher nor the authors, contributors, or editors, assume any liability for any injury and/or damage to persons or property as a matter of products liability, negligence or otherwise, or from any use or operation of any methods, products, instructions, or ideas contained in the material herein.

your source for books,
journals and multimedia
in the health sciences

www.elsevierhealth.com

Working together
to grow libraries in
developing countries

www.elsevier.com • www.bookaid.org

The publisher's policy is to use paper manufactured from sustainable forests

Printed in China

Senior Content Strategist: Pauline Graham
Senior Content Development Specialist: Ailsa Laing
Project Manager: Anne Collett
Designer: Miles Hitchen

Contents

List of abbreviations

5-ASA	5-aminosalicylic acid	DNA	Deoxyribonucleic acid
5-HT	5-hydroxytryptamine (serotonin)	DVT	Deep vein thrombosis
		ECF	Extracellular fluid
ACE	Angiotensin-converting enzyme	ECG	Electrocardiogram
		EEG	Electroencephalography
ACS	Acute coronary syndrome	eGFR	Estimated glomerular filtration rate
ACTH	Adrenocorticotropic hormone		
ADP	Adenosine diphosphate	ENaC	Epithelial sodium channels
AF	Atrial fibrillation	FBC	Full blood count
ALS	Advanced Life Support	FH4	Tetrahydrofolate
ALT	Alanine aminotransferase/ transaminase	FSH	Follicle-stimulating hormone
		G	Gauge
AMP	Adenosine monophosphate	g	Gram
APTR	Activated partial thromboplastin ratio	G6PD	Glucose-6-phosphate dehydrogenase
ARB	Angiotensin receptor blocker	GABA	Gamma-aminobutyric acid
AT_1	Angiotensin type 1 (receptor)	G-CSF	Granulocyte colony stimulating factor
ATP	Adenosine triphosphate		
AV	Atrioventricular	GFR	Glomerular filtration rate
BCG	Bacillus Calmette–Guérin	GI	Gastrointestinal
BMI	Body mass index	GLP-1	Glucagon-like peptide-1
BNF	British National Formulary	GMP	Guanosine monophosphate
BP	Blood pressure	GORD	Gastro-oesophageal reflux disease
Ca^{2+}	Calcium ion		
cGMP	Cyclic guanosine monophosphate	GP	General practitioner
		GTN	Glyceryl trinitrate
CHC	Combined hormonal contraception	H^+	Hydrogen ion
		HAS	Human albumin solution
CKD	Chronic kidney disease	HIV	Human immunodeficiency virus
Cl^-	Chloride ion		
CNS	Central nervous system	HMG	3-hydroxy-3-methyl-glutaryl coenzyme A
CO_2	Carbon dioxide		
COC	Combined oral contraceptive	hr	Hour
COPD	Chronic obstructive pulmonary disease	hrly	Hourly
		HRT	Hormone replacement therapy
COX	Cyclooxygenase		
CPR	Cardiopulmonary resuscitation	HUS	Haemolytic–uraemic syndrome
CT	Computerised tomography	IBS	Irritable bowel syndrome
CTZ	Chemoreceptor trigger zone	Ig	Immunoglobulin
DEXA	Dual-energy X-ray absorptiometry	IL	Interleukin
		IM	Intramuscular
DMARD	Disease-modifying antirheumatic drug	INR	International normalised ratio
		IQ	Intelligence quotient

IR	Immediate-release	NOAC	Novel oral anticoagulant
ISMN	Isosorbide mononitrate	NPH	Neutral protamine Hagedorn
IV	Intravenous	NRT	Nicotine replacement therapy
K^+	Potassium ion	NSAID	Non-steroidal anti-inflammatory drug
kg	Kilogram		
L	Litre	p	Pence
LABA	Long-acting β_2-agonist	PCR	Polymerase chain reaction
LAMA	Long-acting antimuscarinic	PD	Pharmacodynamic
LDL	Low density lipoprotein	PDE	Phosphodiesterase
L-dopa	Levodopa	PGE_2	Prostaglandin
LH	Luteinising hormone	PK	Pharmacokinetic
LMWH	Low molecular weight heparin	PPI	Proton pump inhibitor
		Q fever	Query fever
LRTI	Lower respiratory tract infection	RNA	Ribonucleic acid
		SA	Sinoatrial
m	Metre	SC	Subcutaneous
MDI	Metered dose inhaler	sec	Second
mg	Milligram	SL	Sublingual
MHRA	Medicines and Healthcare products Regulatory Agency	SNRI	Serotonin and noradrenaline reuptake inhibitor
Min	Minute	SSRI	Selective serotonin reuptake inhibitor
mL	Millilitre		
mmHg	Millimetres of mercury	SVT	Supraventricular tachycardia
mmol	Millimole	T_3	Triiodothyronine
MMR	Measles, mumps and rubella	T_4	Thyroxine
MR	Modified release	TNF	Tumour necrosis factor
MRSA	Meticillin-resistant *Staphylococcus aureus*	TSH	Thyroid stimulating hormone
		UC	Ulcerative colitis
mV	Millivolt	UFH	Unfractionated heparin
Na^+	Sodium ion	UK	United Kingdom
NAPQI	N-acetyl-p-benzoquinone imine	UTI	Urinary tract infection
		VF	Ventricular fibrillation
NHS	National Health Service	VT	Ventricular tachycardia
NMS	Neuroleptic malignant syndrome	VTE	Venous thromboembolism
		WHO	World Health Organization

Introduction

Why should you use this book?

Learning pharmacology is hard. In the UK, nearly 2000 drugs are available in over 20,000 medicinal products. The amount of information you could obtain for each one is almost limitless, as is reflected in the hefty weight of conventional pharmacology textbooks. Compounding this, medical schools have recently – and quite appropriately in our view – begun to emphasise the importance of practical prescribing in their curricula and examinations. The classic pharmacology texts that once provided students with all they needed to know (and usually much more) now appear deficient in this critically important area. Meanwhile, the prescribing manuals and formularies used by doctors are generally impenetrable to students, and provide insufficient detail on the clinical pharmacology that underpins the use and understanding of drugs.

Against this backdrop, you need a place to start. You need to focus most of your attention on the most important information about the most important drugs. You need a bridge between a medical student's textbook and a prescriber's manual. Fundamentally, you need to know what you need to know about the drugs you are going to prescribe in practice. That is what this book seeks to provide.

What are 'the top 100 drugs'?

We analysed data from hundreds of millions of prescriptions in primary and secondary care to identify the drugs that were prescribed most often.[1] To this list we added a handful of 'emergency drugs' which, although less commonly used, are important to know about. We tested the stability of the resulting 'top 100' list over the next two years to confirm it did not change significantly. We surveyed 149 foundation doctors who told us that, on average, they prescribed 41 of the top 100 drugs at least every week and another 24 at least every month. More than three-quarters said they rarely prescribed drugs that are not on the list.

How to use this book

Organisation of the book

The top 100 drugs are arranged in alphabetical order. We have generally identified them by the name of the class to which they belong: thus 'bisoprolol' is found under 'beta-blockers'. We have listed common examples in order of the frequency with which they are used, with less common but still important drugs added to this where appropriate. Where a drug is effectively in a class of its own, we have identified it simply by its name: thus we use 'metformin' rather than 'biguanides'. In addition to the top 100 drugs, we have provided details of five commonly used fluid preparations in their own section at the end of the book.

To help you test and reinforce your knowledge, we have included some single-best-answer questions. The answers to these direct you to the relevant drug entries as appropriate. These also provide an opportunity to bring together information from several drugs and show how it may be integrated in practice.

Using the book

We anticipate this book being used in two main ways. One is as a 'quick reference source' for when you encounter a drug on the ward or in clinic and want to read

Table 1.1   Anatomy of the 'drug' pages

Drug class (or drug name, if it is in a class of its own)

CLINICAL PHARMACOLOGY

Common indications	A list of the **situations in which the drug is commonly used**, along with brief discussion of its **place in therapy;** in other words, where it fits in alongside other treatment options.
Mechanism of action	A brief discussion of how the drug works in the indications specified.
Important adverse effects	The most common and important adverse effects of the drug, with discussion of their mechanism where this aids understanding.
Warnings	The situations in which the drug should be avoided (i.e. is **contraindicated**) or where extra **caution** should be used.
Important interactions	The most important interactions with other drugs.

up on it quickly. The alphabetical arrangement of the drugs aims to facilitate this. The other way you might use it is when learning about an organ system or a disease and want core information about the relevant drugs. To support this way of working, we have provided two additional tables of contents: one listing the drugs relevant to each system, and the other listing drugs used in specific indications.

In your early years at medical school, you will probably concentrate on learning clinical pharmacology. As you progress, you will increasingly need to supplement this with knowledge and skills in practical prescribing. Reflecting this, we have arranged the information under these two main headings in a consistent way throughout the book. We have further divided the information with standard subheadings, the purpose of which is outlined in Table 1.1. We use bold text and icons to draw out key points, as indicated in Box 1.1.

Using the information

We provide information that we hope will inform your understanding of drugs and their practical use, but this is not a prescribing formulary. This is particularly important in relation to cautions and contraindications (which we refer to collectively as 'warnings'). To reproduce all the points that might need to be considered in practice would be overwhelming and destroy the point of the book. Likewise for drug doses, we will often provide a 'typical starting dose' because we think it's useful for you to have an idea of the kind of doses you will see used in practice. However, it is not our intention that when writing real prescriptions you will look up doses in this book. The key point is this: this book is for *learning*. When you start

Common examples, in order of relative importance

PRACTICAL PRESCRIBING

Prescription	A discussion of how the drug is usually prescribed including, as appropriate, typical starting dosage and route of administration.
Administration	A discussion of any important considerations about how the drug should be administered, beyond those already covered by the prescription.
Communication	A brief discussion of the important information that should be conveyed to the patient, written in non-medical language.
Monitoring	Details about how the efficacy and safety of treatment should be monitored.
Cost	A brief mention of cost, particularly to highlight where savings can be made without affecting treatment efficacy.

Clinical tip—an interesting or useful fact or tip about the drug, generally derived from clinical experience.

Box 1.1 Text features used throughout the book

Bold text is used to highlight key points for quick identification.

<u>Underlining</u> is used to identify drugs that are covered elsewhere in the book in more detail.

A ▲ **red triangle** is used to identify important circumstances such as comorbidities (cautions and contraindications) or concurrent medications (interactions) in which use of the drug is risky. Although it may occasionally be used, this would be appropriate only after careful risk–benefit assessment and some extra safety measures, such as lower dosage and more intensive monitoring. As a foundation doctor, you would generally be expected to seek senior or specialist guidance in these situations.

A ✖ **red cross** is used to identify circumstances (such as comorbidities or concurrent medications) in which we regard use of the drug to be dangerous and inappropriate.

making decisions for patients, you will need to consult a formulary (in the UK, the *British National Formulary* [BNF]). You can practise this now – the knowledge you will acquire from this book will make the BNF more useful and accessible.

Where next?

This book provides, in our judgement, the most important information that you need to know about drugs in order to pass your examinations and, ultimately, to become a safe and effective foundation doctor. However, in providing you with this 'starting point', it is not our intention to stifle your inquisitiveness. We would actively encourage you to learn more, both about the drugs in this book and others that are less commonly used. We just know, from many years' experience teaching doctors and students, that when confronted with such an overwhelming number of drugs, and all the things you could possibly know about them, it is sometimes difficult to see the wood for the trees.

Reference

1. Baker EH *et al*. Development of a core drug list towards improving prescribing education and reducing errors in the UK. *British Journal of Clinical Pharmacology* 2011;71:190–198.

The top 100 drugs listed by system

The top 100 drugs listed by indication

Acne	Tetracyclines	200
Acute coronary syndrome	Angiotensin-converting enzyme (ACE) inhibitors	44
	Aspirin	78
	Beta-blockers	84
	Clopidogrel	96
	Fibrinolytic drugs	120
	Heparins and fondaparinux	126
	Nitrates	154
	Opioids, strong	166
	Statins	196
Addison's disease	Corticosteroids (glucocorticoids), systemic	100
Adrenal insufficiency	Corticosteroids (glucocorticoids), systemic	100
Agitation, psychomotor	Antiemetics, phenothiazines	58
	Antipsychotics, first-generation (typical)	74
	Antipsychotics, second-generation (atypical)	76
Alcohol withdrawal	Benzodiazepines	80
Allergy	Antihistamines (H_1-receptor antagonists)	64
	Corticosteroids (glucocorticoids), systemic	100
Anaemia	Iron	130
	Vitamins	214
Anaphylaxis	Adrenaline (epinephrine)	28
	Antihistamines (H_1-receptor antagonists)	64
	Corticosteroids (glucocorticoids), systemic	100
Angina	Beta-blockers	84
	Calcium channel blockers	90
	Nicorandil	150
	Nitrates	154
Anxiety	Antidepressants, selective serotonin reuptake inhibitors	48
	Antidepressants, venlafaxine and mirtazepine	52
	Benzodiazepines	80
	Gabapentin and pregabalin	122

The top 100 drugs

Acetylcysteine (N-acetylcysteine)

CLINICAL PHARMACOLOGY

Common indications	❶ As the antidote for **paracetamol poisoning.** ❷ To help prevent renal injury due to radiographic contrast material **(contrast nephropathy).** ❸ To reduce the viscosity of **respiratory secretions** (acting as a mucolytic).
Mechanisms of action	In therapeutic doses, <u>paracetamol</u> is metabolised mainly by conjugation with glucuronic acid and sulfate. A small amount is converted to N-acetyl-p-benzoquinone imine (NAPQI), which is hepatotoxic. Normally, this is quickly detoxified by conjugation with glutathione. However, in paracetamol poisoning, the body's supply of glutathione is overwhelmed and NAPQI is left free to cause liver damage. Acetylcysteine works mainly by **replenishing the body's supply of glutathione.** Acetylcysteine also has antioxidant effects, which may contribute to its effect in preventing contrast nephropathy, although this is not completely understood. If acetylcysteine is brought into contact with mucus, it causes it to liquefy. For patients who have tenacious respiratory secretions (e.g. in bronchiectasis), this may aid sputum clearance.
Important adverse effects	When administered intravenously in large doses for paracetamol poisoning, acetylcysteine can cause an **anaphylactoid reaction.** This is similar to an anaphylactic reaction (presenting with nausea, tachycardia, rash and wheeze), but involves histamine release independent of IgE antibodies. Therefore, once the reaction has settled (by stopping the acetylcysteine and giving an antihistamine ± a bronchodilator), it is usually safe to restart acetylcysteine, but at a lower rate of infusion. When administered in nebulised form as a mucolytic, acetylcysteine may cause **bronchospasm.** Therefore, a bronchodilator (e.g. <u>salbutamol</u>) should usually be given immediately beforehand.
Warnings	History of an anaphylactoid reaction to acetylcysteine does not contraindicate its use in future, if it is required. It is important that such reactions are not labelled as 'allergic,' which may lead to effective treatment for paracetamol poisoning being inappropriately denied. However, it is essential to obtain specialist advice if there is any doubt.
Important interactions	There are no significant adverse drug interactions with acetylcysteine.

acetylcysteine

PRACTICAL PRESCRIBING

Prescription	In the treatment of **paracetamol poisoning,** weight-adjusted doses are given as an IV infusion with three components (total infusion time 21 hours). You should consult the BNF and/or a local protocol for full details. For use in the prophylaxis of **contrast nephropathy,** you should consult local guidelines as dosing instructions may not be given in the BNF. The usual dose is 600–1200 mg orally 12-hrly for 2 days, beginning the day before the procedure. For use in tenacious **respiratory secretions,** a typical dose is 2.5–5 mL of acetylcysteine 10% solution by nebuliser every 6 hours, but again, you should follow local protocols.
Administration	Detailed instructions for the preparation and administration of acetylcysteine in paracetamol poisoning are provided in a technical information leaflet that is provided with the product and is also available online. For use as a mucolytic, the 20% intravenous solution should be diluted to a 10% solution before use.
Communication	Explain that you are offering treatment with a paracetamol antidote. It is given slowly through a drip over 21 hours. If it is started within about 8 hours of a single overdose, you can say that it is very effective and, provided it is administered correctly, should completely prevent serious damage to the liver. Emphasise the importance of avoiding interruptions to the treatment, while acknowledging the inconvenience of being 'tied to a drip' for the best part of a day. Mention that it occasionally causes a reaction involving a rash, nausea, or wheeziness. They should alert staff if they notice any of these symptoms, so that the infusion can be interrupted and treatment given.
Monitoring	In the treatment of paracetamol poisoning, patients should be monitored clinically for signs of anaphylactoid reaction. The international normalised ratio (INR), serum alanine aminotransferase (ALT) activity and creatinine concentration should be measured at presentation and on completion of the acetylcysteine. The INR is the most sensitive marker of ongoing liver injury and recovery of liver function in this situation.
Cost	Acetylcysteine is available in non-proprietary form and is relatively inexpensive.

Clinical tip—The UK guidelines for the use of acetylcysteine in paracetamol poisoning changed in 2012. These changes affected both who should be treated and how it should be administered. Make sure you refer to material produced from 2012 onwards in order to obtain the correct information.

Activated charcoal

CLINICAL PHARMACOLOGY

Common indications	❶ A *single dose* of activated charcoal may be used to **reduce absorption** of **certain poisons** (including some **drugs in overdose**) from the gut. ❷ *Multiple doses* of activated charcoal may also be used to **increase the elimination** of **certain poisons.**
Mechanisms of action	Van der Waals (weak intermolecular) forces are responsible for the mechanism of action of activated charcoal. **Molecules are *ad*sorbed onto the surface of the charcoal** as they travel through the gut, **reducing their *ab*sorption** into the circulation. However, activated charcoal is only useful in cases where the poison ingested is likely to be adsorbed onto it. The affinity of a substance for activated charcoal is determined by its ionic status and its solubility in water. Weakly ionic, hydrophobic substances (e.g. benzodiazepines, methotrexate) are generally well adsorbed to activated charcoal. By contrast, strongly ionic and hydrophilic substances (e.g. strong acids/bases, alcohols, lithium and iron) are not adsorbed. Activated charcoal can also **increase the elimination** of certain poisons. This may be useful for substances adsorbed by charcoal that can **readily diffuse back into the gut.** In this case, multiple doses of activated charcoal can be used to maintain a steep concentration gradient of the poison (high in the circulation, low in the gut), encouraging diffusion out of the circulation and hastening elimination of the drug. This is sometimes referred to as 'gut dialysis'. Of note, charcoal is 'activated' during preparation through chemical processes, including blasting it with steam or hot air. These processes increase the surface area of the charcoal particles by increasing pore size. With a surface area around 1000 m^2/g, a lot of poison can be adsorbed!
Important adverse effects	**Aspiration** of activated charcoal can lead to serious complications such as **pneumonitis, bronchospasm** and **airway obstruction.** It can also precipitate **intestinal obstruction.** However, the most common adverse effects of activated charcoal are **black stools** and **vomiting.**
Warnings	Activated charcoal should not be used in patients with a ▲**reduced level of consciousness,** unless their airway is first protected by endotracheal intubation. Caution is required when prescribing activated charcoal to patients with ▲**persistent vomiting,** as there is a risk of aspiration. Those with ▲**reduced gastrointestinal motility** have an increased risk of intestinal obstruction.
Important interactions	Activated charcoal prevents absorption of many drugs taken therapeutically as well as those taken in overdose.

PRACTICAL PRESCRIBING

Prescription	A *single dose* of activated charcoal to reduce absorption is recommended only for patients presenting **within 1 hour of ingestion of a clinically significant amount of a substance that is adsorbed by charcoal.** For drugs that delay gastric emptying (e.g. aspirin, opioids, tricyclic antidepressants), charcoal can be administered up to 2 hours following ingestion. Activated charcoal should be prescribed on the once-only section of the drug chart at a dose of 50 g orally (or by nasogastric tube if the patient is intubated). When using *multiple doses* of activated charcoal (potential situations include significant overdose with carbamazepine, quinine, or theophylline – but seek advice), you should prescribe 50 g of activated charcoal to be administered 4-hrly. Pre-emptive treatment with an antiemetic and a laxative may be advisable.
Administration	Activated charcoal is usually mixed with 250 mL of water to form a suspension, which the patient then drinks. In patients who are unconscious but have a protected airway (i.e. following intubation), this suspension may be given via a nasogastric tube.
Communication	Advise patients that activated charcoal can help prevent absorption of the drug or poison they have taken. It may also be worth mentioning that the taste is not particularly palatable!
Monitoring	No special monitoring is necessary when a patient takes activated charcoal above that required for the overdose/poisoning situation.
Cost	A single dose of activated charcoal costs around £12.

Clinical tip—If your patient has vomited prior to presentation, but it is still felt that activated charcoal would be useful, give an antiemetic such as ondansetron (4–8 mg IV) or cyclizine (50 mg IV or IM). However, remember that if the patient is *actively vomiting*, the charcoal may not be effective (as it will not remain in the gastrointestinal tract) and there is a risk of aspiration (see Important adverse effects above).

Adenosine

CLINICAL PHARMACOLOGY

Common indications	❶ As a first-line diagnostic and therapeutic agent in **supraventricular tachycardia (SVT).**
Mechanisms of action	Adenosine is an agonist of adenosine receptors on cell surfaces. In the heart, activation of these G protein-coupled receptors induces a number of effects, including reducing the frequency of spontaneous depolarisations (automaticity) and increasing resistance to depolarisation (refractoriness). In turn, this transiently slows the sinus rate, conduction velocity, and **increases atrioventricular (AV) node refractoriness.** Many forms of SVT arise from a self-perpetuating electrical (re-entry) circuit that takes in the AV node. Increasing refractoriness in the AV node **breaks the re-entry circuit,** which allows normal depolarisations from the sinoatrial (SA) node to resume control of heart rate (**cardioversion**). Where the circuit does not involve the AV node (e.g. in atrial flutter), adenosine will not induce cardioversion. However, by blocking conduction to the ventricles, it allows closer inspection of the atrial rhythm on the ECG. This may reveal the diagnosis. The duration of effect of adenosine is very short because it is rapidly taken up by cells (e.g. red cells). Its half-life in plasma is less than 10 seconds.
Important adverse effects	By interfering with the functions of the SA and AV nodes, adenosine can induce **bradycardia** and even **asystole.** Inevitably, this is accompanied by a deeply unpleasant sensation for the patient. It is said to feel like a **sinking feeling** in the chest, often accompanied by **breathlessness** and a **sense of 'impending doom.'** Fortunately, due to the drug's short-lived effect, this feeling is only brief.
Warnings	You should not administer adenosine to a patient who will not tolerate its transient bradycardic effects, including those with ✖**hypotension,** ✖**coronary ischaemia,** or ✖**decompensated heart failure.** Adenosine may induce bronchospasm in susceptible individuals, so should be avoided in patients with ✖**asthma** or ▲**COPD.** Patients who have had a ▲**heart transplant** are very sensitive to the effects of adenosine.
Important interactions	▲Dipyridamole blocks cellular uptake of adenosine, which prolongs and potentiates its effect: the dose of adenosine should be halved. Theophylline, aminophylline and caffeine are competitive antagonists of adenosine receptors and reduce its effect. Patients who have taken these drugs respond poorly and may require higher doses.

PRACTICAL PRESCRIBING

Prescription	Adenosine is always given intravenously. The prescription should be written in the once-only section of the drug chart. The initial dose is usually 6 mg IV. If this is ineffective, a 12 mg dose may be given. Higher doses may be given in selected cases. If using a central line, lower doses should be used (e.g. 3 mg initially).
Administration	Adenosine should be administered only by a doctor experienced in its use, or under their direct supervision. **Resuscitation facilities** should be on hand. It is important that the adenosine dose reaches the heart quickly to minimise cellular uptake *en route*. This requires a **large-bore cannula** (e.g. 18 gauge [green] or bigger), sited as proximally as possible (e.g. in the antecubital fossa). Administer the dose as a **rapid injection** and then immediately follow it with a flush, e.g. 20 mL of 0.9% sodium chloride. The effect will usually be evident on the cardiac monitor within 10–15 seconds, and then dissipate over about 30–60 seconds.
Communication	Explain that you are offering treatment with a medicine that will hopefully 'reset' their heart into a normal rhythm. Explain that it will briefly make them feel terrible, but this sensation will only last for about 30 seconds. Ensure you continue talking to the patient during its administration, offering reassurance that the unpleasant sensation will go away quickly. Observing profound bradycardia or transient asystole on the cardiac monitor will probably induce some anxiety on your part too. Try not to convey this to the patient!
Monitoring	Administration of adenosine requires very close monitoring. This *must* include a **continuous cardiac rhythm strip,** recorded for subsequent examination.
Cost	Adenosine is inexpensive.

Clinical tip—Advance preparation is invaluable in the administration of adenosine. Plan what doses you will give and draw these up away from the bedside. Use small syringes (e.g. 2 mL) for adenosine, as this will make it easier to administer rapidly. Draw up one 20 mL 0.9% sodium chloride flush for each planned dose, plus one 'spare'. *Label all the syringes carefully.* To administer the drug, first attach a three-way tap to the cannula. Use your 'spare' flush to check its patency. Next, replace this with a new, full 20 mL flush, and attach the first dose of adenosine to the other port. Start the continuous ECG trace, then (after warning the patient) administer the adenosine and the flush in rapid succession. Write the dose administered on the ECG paper as it comes out of the machine.

Adrenaline (epinephrine)

CLINICAL PHARMACOLOGY

Common indications	❶ In **cardiac arrest,** adrenaline is routinely administered as part of the Advanced Life Support (ALS) treatment algorithm. ❷ In **anaphylaxis,** adrenaline is a vital part of immediate management. ❸ Adrenaline may be injected directly into tissues to induce **local vasoconstriction.** For example, it is used during endoscopy to **control mucosal bleeding,** and it is sometimes mixed with local anaesthetic drugs (e.g. <u>lidocaine</u>) to **prolong local anaesthesia.**
Mechanisms of action	Adrenaline is a **potent agonist of the α_1, α_2, β_1 and β_2 adrenoceptors,** and correspondingly has a multitude of sympathetic ('fight or flight') effects. These include: vasoconstriction of vessels supplying skin, mucosa and abdominal viscera (mainly α_1-mediated); increases in heart rate, force of contraction and myocardial excitability (β_1); and vasodilatation of vessels supplying the heart and muscles (β_2). These explain its use in cardiac arrest, where the **redistribution of blood flow in favour of the heart** is desirable, at least theoretically, and may improve the chances of restoring an organised rhythm. Additional effects of adrenaline, mediated by β_2 receptors, are **bronchodilatation and suppression of inflammatory mediator release from mast cells.** Together with its vascular effects, these underpin its use in anaphylaxis, where widespread release of inflammatory mediators from mast cells produces generalised vasodilatation, profound hypotension and often bronchoconstriction.
Important adverse effects	Adrenaline is a dangerous drug, but its risks are balanced against the severity of the condition being treated. In cardiac arrest, restoration of output is often followed by **adrenaline-induced hypertension.** When given to conscious patients in anaphylaxis or in an attempt to produce local vasoconstriction, it often causes **anxiety, tremor, headache** and **palpitations.** It may also cause **angina, myocardial infarction** and **arrhythmias,** particularly in patients with existing heart disease.
Warnings	There are **no contraindications to its use in cardiac arrest and anaphylaxis.** When given to induce local vasoconstriction, it should be used with caution in patients with ▲**heart disease.** Combination adrenaline–anaesthetic preparations should not be used in ✖**areas supplied by an end-artery** (i.e. with poor collateral supply), such as fingers and toes, where vasoconstriction can cause tissue necrosis.
Important interactions	In patients receiving treatment with a ▲<u>β-blocker</u>, adrenaline may induce widespread vasoconstriction, because its α_1-mediated vasoconstricting effect is not opposed by β_2-mediated vasodilatation.

PRACTICAL PRESCRIBING

Prescription	In life-threatening situations, adrenaline is administered first then prescribed later. In adult **cardiac arrest** associated with a shockable rhythm (ventricular fibrillation or pulseless ventricular tachycardia), adrenaline 1 mg IV is given just after the third shock, and repeated every 3–5 minutes thereafter (i.e. every other cycle of CPR). If the rhythm is not shockable (asystole or pulseless electrical activity), adrenaline 1 mg IV is given as soon as IV access is available, and then repeated every 3–5 minutes. In **anaphylaxis,** the dose of adrenaline is 500 micrograms IM, repeated after 5 minutes if necessary. Take particular note of the route of administration: **do not administer IV adrenaline in anaphylaxis, unless cardiac arrest supervenes.** When administered with a local anaesthetic to induce **local vasoconstriction,** a ready-mixed adrenaline–anaesthetic preparation should be used; usually this contains adrenaline at a concentration of 1:200,000 (5 micrograms/mL) along with the anaesthetic. The name 'adrenaline' is still used for prescribing in the UK, although the international non-proprietary name (epinephrine) is also printed on product packaging.
Administration	In **cardiac arrest,** adrenaline is administered from a pre-filled syringe containing a 1:10,000 (1 mg in 10 mL) solution. Administer the whole 10 mL, followed by a flush (e.g. 10 mL of 0.9% sodium chloride). In **anaphylaxis,** give 0.5 mL of a 1:1000 (1 mg in 1 mL) adrenaline solution by IM injection. Inject this into the anterolateral aspect of the thigh halfway between the knee and the hip, from where it should be rapidly absorbed. In obese patients you need to inject deeply in order to be confident of IM rather than SC administration.
Communication	In **anaphylaxis,** simultaneously with providing treatment, explain to the patient that they are experiencing a severe allergic reaction and that you are giving them an injection of adrenaline to treat this.
Monitoring	In the context of **cardiac arrest** and **anaphylaxis,** intensive clinical and haemodynamic monitoring is essential.
Cost	Cost is not relevant to decisions regarding the use of adrenaline.

Clinical tip—The use of a local anaesthetic mixed with adrenaline often induces a mild but quite unpleasant sensation of anxiety for the patient. This only adds to the tension associated with undergoing a procedure. The use of adrenaline in this context is probably most appropriate in the operating theatre, where it can be injected while the patient is under general anaesthesia as a means of prolonging post-operative analgesia.

Aldosterone antagonists

CLINICAL PHARMACOLOGY

Common indications	❶ **Ascites and oedema due to liver cirrhosis:** spironolactone is the first-line diuretic. ❷ **Chronic heart failure:** of at least moderate severity or arising within 1 month of a myocardial infarction, usually as an addition to a β-blocker and an <u>ACE inhibitor</u>/<u>angiotensin receptor blocker</u>. ❸ **Primary hyperaldosteronism:** for patients awaiting surgery or for whom surgery is not an option.
Mechanisms of action	Aldosterone is a mineralocorticoid that is produced in the adrenal cortex. It acts on mineralocorticoid receptors in the distal tubules of the kidney to increase the activity of luminal epithelial sodium channels (ENaC). This increases the reabsorption of sodium and water (which elevates blood pressure) with the by-product of increased potassium excretion. Aldosterone antagonists inhibit the effect of aldosterone by **competitively binding to the aldosterone receptor.** This increases sodium and water excretion and potassium retention. Their effect is greatest in primary hyperaldosteronism or when circulating aldosterone is increased, e.g. in cirrhosis.
Important adverse effects	An important adverse effect of aldosterone antagonists is **hyperkalaemia,** which can lead to muscle weakness, arrhythmias and even cardiac arrest. Spironolactone causes **gynaecomastia,** which can have a significant impact on patient adherence (see Communication). Aldosterone antagonists can cause liver impairment and jaundice and are a cause of Stevens–Johnson syndrome (a T cell-mediated hypersensitivity reaction) that causes a bullous skin eruption.
Warnings	Aldosterone antagonists are contraindicated in patients with ✖**severe renal impairment,** ✖**hyperkalaemia** and ✖**Addison's disease** (who are aldosterone deficient). Aldosterone antagonists can cross the placenta during pregnancy and appear in breast milk so should be avoided where possible in ▲**pregnant or lactating women.**
Important interactions	The combination of an aldosterone antagonist with other ▲**potassium-elevating drugs,** including ▲<u>ACE inhibitors</u> and ▲<u>angiotensin receptor blockers</u>, increases the risk of hyperkalaemia. Nevertheless, when supported by appropriate monitoring, this may be a beneficial combination in the context of heart failure. Aldosterone antagonists should not be combined with ✖<u>potassium supplements</u> except in specialist practice.

PRACTICAL PRESCRIBING

Prescription	Aldosterone antagonists are only available as oral preparations. Spironolactone is used for all indications, whereas eplerenone is only licensed for the treatment of heart failure. Aldosterone antagonists should be prescribed for regular administration, generally as a single daily dose. You should tailor the dose to the specific indication as, for example, much higher doses are used to treat ascites secondary to cirrhosis than are used in heart failure. A typical starting dose of spironolactone is 100 mg daily for ascites compared to 25 mg daily for heart failure. Spironolactone is also available as a combined preparation with a thiazide or loop diuretic.
Administration	Spironolactone should generally be taken with food.
Communication	When starting treatment with spironolactone, particularly in high doses, it is particularly important to warn men about the possibility of **growth and tenderness of tissue under the nipples** and **impotence.** Reassure them that such effects are benign and reversible, but acknowledge that they may be uncomfortable and embarrassing. Ask patients to return if they have troublesome side effects, as these may respond to dose reduction. Advise all patients that aldosterone antagonists can cause their potassium level to rise and reinforce the importance of attending for blood tests.
Monitoring	**Efficacy** should be monitored by patient report of symptoms and clinical findings, e.g. reduction in ascites, oedema and/or blood pressure. **Safety** should be monitored by checking renal function and serum potassium concentration due to risk of renal impairment and hyperkalaemia.
Cost	Spironolactone is available in non-proprietary form and costs about £1.50 per month, whereas eplerenone is still protected by patent and costs about £40 per month.

Clinical tip—Spironolactone is a relatively weak diuretic that takes several days to start having an effect. It is therefore usually prescribed in combination with a loop or thiazide diuretic, where it both counteracts potassium wasting and potentiates the diuretic effect. For example, in the treatment of ascites due to chronic liver failure, spironolactone and furosemide are generally used together in a ratio of about 5:1 (e.g. spironolactone 200 mg with furosemide 40 mg).

Alginates and antacids

CLINICAL PHARMACOLOGY

Common indications	❶ **Gastro-oesophageal reflux disease:** for symptomatic relief of heartburn. ❷ **Dyspepsia:** for short-term relief of indigestion.
Mechanisms of action	These drugs are most often taken as compound preparations containing an alginate with one or more antacids, such as sodium bicarbonate, calcium carbonate, magnesium or aluminium salts. *Antacids* work by **buffering** stomach acids. *Alginates* act to increase the **viscosity** of the stomach contents, which reduces the reflux of stomach acid into the oesophagus. After reacting with stomach acid they form a floating **'raft'**, which separates the gastric contents from the gastro-oesophageal junction to prevent mucosal damage. There is some evidence to suggest they also inhibit pepsin production. Antacids alone (usually aluminium or magnesium compounds) can be used for the short-term relief of dyspepsia.
Important adverse effects	Compound alginates cause few side effects, which vary depending on their constituents and the dose taken. Magnesium salts can cause **diarrhoea,** whereas aluminium salts can cause **constipation.**
Warnings	Compound alginates are well tolerated and are safe in pregnancy. Paediatric formulations are safe for use in infants, but compound alginates should not be given in combination with ▲**thickened milk preparations** as they can lead to excessively thick stomach contents that cause bloating and abdominal discomfort. Sodium- and potassium-containing preparations should be used with caution in patients with fluid overload or hyperkalaemia (e.g. ▲**renal failure**). Some preparations contain sucrose, which can worsen hyperglycaemia in people with diabetes mellitus.
Important interactions	The divalent cations in compound alginates can bind to other drugs, reducing their absorption. Antacids can reduce serum concentrations of many drugs, so the doses should be taken at different times. This applies to ACE inhibitors, some antibiotics (e.g. cephalosporins, ciprofloxacin and tetracyclines), bisphosphonates, digoxin, levothyroxine and proton pump inhibitors. By increasing the alkalinity of urine, antacids can increase the excretion of aspirin and lithium.

PRACTICAL PRESCRIBING

Prescription	Compound alginates are available as oral suspension or chewable tablets. Only proprietary compound alginates are available, therefore you can prescribe by brand name. They are usually prescribed as required for symptomatic relief. Check the constituents of the brand chosen, particularly if prescribing for patients with renal impairment or diabetes mellitus.
Administration	They should be taken following meals, before bedtime and/or when symptoms occur. For infants, oral powder can be mixed with feeds or water.
Communication	Explain that the medicine should relieve the symptoms of heartburn and acid indigestion within about 20 minutes and for several hours afterwards. However, advise that this is only a temporary measure. Discuss **lifestyle measures** that can be taken to reduce reflux, such as eating smaller meals more often, identifying and avoiding food and drink triggers, stopping smoking and raising the head of the bed. Warn patients to return for review if symptoms persist. Advise patients to take compound alginates after mealtimes and before bed. Advise them to **leave a gap of at least 2 hours** between these medicines and other drugs that they may intact with (see Interactions).
Monitoring	Symptomatic response should be monitored by the patient and their healthcare practitioner. If there are persistent symptoms or 'red flags', such as bleeding, vomiting, dysphagia and weight loss, then further investigation and specialist review should be considered.
Cost	Compound alginates are inexpensive. They can be purchased over the counter. If prescribing, you should prescribe the lowest cost brand available.

Clinical tip—Compound alginates are a useful treatment in the armamentarium of the paediatrician. Around 10–20% of children suffer from gastro-oesophageal reflux disease, and compound alginates have been shown to reduce frequency of symptoms.

Allopurinol

CLINICAL PHARMACOLOGY

Common indications	❶ To prevent acute attacks of **gout.** ❷ To prevent uric acid and calcium oxalate **renal stones.** ❸ To prevent **hyperuricaemia** and **tumour lysis syndrome** associated with chemotherapy.
Mechanisms of action	Allopurinol is a **xanthine oxidase inhibitor**. Xanthine oxidase metabolises xanthine (produced from purines) to uric acid. Inhibition of xanthine oxidase lowers plasma uric acid concentrations and reduces precipitation of uric acid in the joints or kidneys.
Important adverse effects	Allopurinol is generally well tolerated. The most common side effect is a **skin rash**, which may be mild or may indicate a more serious hypersensitivity reaction such as **Stevens–Johnson syndrome** or **toxic epidermal necrolysis. Drug hypersensitivity syndrome** is a rare, life-threatening reaction to allopurinol that can include fever, eosinophilia, lymphadenopathy and involvement of other organs, such as the liver and skin. Starting allopurinol can **trigger or worsen an acute attack of gout.**
Warnings	Allopurinol should not be started during ✖**acute attacks of gout,** but can be continued if a patient is already established on it, to avoid sudden fluctuations in serum uric acid levels. ✖**Recurrent skin rash** or signs of more ✖**severe hypersensitivity** to allopurinol are contraindications to therapy. Allopurinol is metabolised in the liver and excreted by the kidney. The dose should therefore be reduced in patients with severe ▲**renal impairment** or ▲**hepatic impairment.**
Important interactions	The cytotoxic drug ▲mercaptopurine and its pro-drug ▲azathioprine require xanthine oxidase for metabolism. When allopurinol is prescribed with these drugs, it inhibits their metabolism and increases the risk of toxicity. Co-prescription of allopurinol with amoxicillin increases the risk of skin rash and with ACE inhibitors or thiazides increases the risk of hypersensitivity reactions.

PRACTICAL PRESCRIBING

Prescription	Allopurinol is taken orally. Start at a low dose (e.g. 100 mg daily) and titrate up according to serum uric acid concentrations to usual maintenance of 200–600 mg daily in 1–2 divided doses. When starting allopurinol **for gout,** NSAID or colchicine treatment should also be prescribed and continued for at least a month after serum uric acid levels return to normal to avoid triggering an acute attack. Although allopurinol should not be started during an acute attack of gout, patients who are already on it should continue to take it. Where allopurinol is used **as part of cancer treatment,** it should be commenced before chemotherapy.
Administration	Allopurinol should be taken after meals and patients should be encouraged to maintain good hydration with fluid intake of 2–3 litres daily.
Communication	Advise patients that the purpose of treatment is to **reduce attacks of gout** (or formation of kidney stones). Warn patients to **seek medical advice if they develop a rash.** Explain that this is usually mild and goes away on stopping the drug, but it can be a sign of a more serious allergy. Advise patients not to stop allopurinol if they get an acute attack of gout, as this could make the attack worse.
Monitoring	Serum uric acid concentrations should be checked 4 weeks after initiating allopurinol or after a change in dose. You should aim to lower uric acid concentrations to less than 300 µmol/L where possible, by increasing the dose of allopurinol as needed. Allopurinol treatment should be **stopped if a rash develops.** For mild skin rashes, treatment can be reintroduced cautiously once the rash resolves. Recurrence of the rash or signs of more severe hypersensitivity to allopurinol are contraindications to further therapy.
Cost	Allopurinol is available in a non-proprietary form and is inexpensive.

Clinical tip—Treatment with thiazide or loop diuretics increases serum uric acid concentrations and can cause gout. Low-dose aspirin inhibits renal excretion of uric acid and can trigger acute attacks of gout. Always consider drug-induced gout as a cause of new-onset joint pain in patients taking these medicines.

Alpha-blockers

CLINICAL PHARMACOLOGY

Common indications	❶ As a first-line medical option to improve symptoms in **benign prostatic hyperplasia,** when lifestyle changes are insufficient. 5α-reductase inhibitors may be added in selected cases. Surgical treatment is also an option, particularly if there is evidence of urinary tract damage (e.g. hydronephrosis). ❷ As an add-on treatment in **resistant hypertension,** when other medicines (e.g. calcium channel blockers, ACE inhibitors, thiazide diuretics) are insufficient.
Mechanisms of action	Although often described using the broad term 'α-blocker,' most drugs in this class (including doxazosin, tamsulosin and alfuzosin) are highly selective for the α_1-adrenoceptor. Alpha$_1$-adrenoceptors are found mainly in smooth muscle, including in blood vessels and the urinary tract (the bladder neck and prostate in particular). Stimulation induces contraction; blockade induces relaxation. Alpha$_1$-blockers therefore cause **vasodilatation** and a fall in blood pressure, and **reduced resistance to bladder outflow.**
Important adverse effects	Predictably from their effects on vascular tone, α-blockers can cause **postural hypotension, dizziness** and **syncope.** This is particularly prominent after the first dose (rather like with ACE inhibitors and angiotensin receptor blockers).
Warnings	Alpha-blockers should not be used in patients with existing ▲**postural hypotension.**
Important interactions	In general, combining antihypertensive drugs results in additive blood pressure lowering effects (this may well be the therapeutic aim). To avoid pronounced first-dose hypotension, it may be prudent to omit doses of one or more existing antihypertensive drugs on the day the α-blocker is started. This is particularly the case for β-blockers, which inhibit the reflex tachycardia that forms part of the compensatory response to vasodilatation.

doxazosin, tamsulosin, alfuzosin

PRACTICAL PRESCRIBING

Prescription	Doxazosin and tamsulosin are the most commonly prescribed α-blockers in the UK. They are taken orally. Doxazosin is licensed both for **benign prostatic hyperplasia** and **hypertension;** it is typically started at a dose of 1 mg daily and increased at 1–2 week intervals according to response. Tamsulosin is only licensed for **benign prostatic hyperplasia.** It also has a blood pressure lowering effect, but this is probably less pronounced than for doxazosin. It is given in a dose of 400 micrograms daily.
Administration	Given the pronounced blood pressure lowering effect of doxazosin, it is best to take this at bedtime, at least initially.
Communication	As appropriate, advise your patient that you are offering them a treatment for their urinary symptoms or their blood pressure. Explain that it may cause dizziness on standing, particularly after the first dose. Advise them to start by taking the medicine at bedtime to minimise the impact of this.
Monitoring	The best guide to **efficacy** is the patient's urinary symptoms and/or blood pressure, as applicable. For **safety,** adverse effects are identified by symptom enquiry and by measuring their lying and standing blood pressure.
Cost	Non-proprietary forms of doxazosin and tamsulosin are inexpensive. Both drugs are also available in modified-release forms which, as brand name products, are more expensive. There is little convincing evidence that the modified-release forms are any more effective than standard-release forms, and since they are all taken at the same frequency (daily), they do not improve convenience for the patient.

Clinical tip—Although in hypertension α-blockers are usually reserved for patients who do not respond to other drug classes, many men with hypertension also have benign prostatic hyperplasia. Discovering that a man with hypertension also has benign prostatic hyperplasia may prompt you to introduce doxazosin at an earlier stage in the treatment pathway. In doing so, you may be able to improve both conditions with a single drug. This exemplifies why the 'review of systems' is an important part of history taking.

Aminoglycosides

CLINICAL PHARMACOLOGY

Common indications	Severe infections, particularly those caused by Gram-negative aerobes (including *Pseudomonas aeruginosa*): ❶ **Severe sepsis,** including where the source is unidentified. ❷ **Pyelonephritis** and **complicated urinary tract infection.** ❸ **Biliary** and other **intra-abdominal sepsis.** ❹ **Endocarditis.** Aminoglycosides lack activity against streptococci and anaerobes (see Mechanisms of action), so should be combined with <u>penicillin</u> and/or <u>metronidazole</u> when the organism is unknown.
Mechanisms of action	Aminoglycosides **bind irreversibly to bacterial ribosomes** (30S subunit) and inhibit protein synthesis. They are bactericidal (i.e. they kill bacteria), although this effect is likely to be due to additional mechanisms that are incompletely understood. Their spectrum of action includes Gram-negative aerobic bacteria, staphylococci and mycobacteria (for example, streptomycin was one of the first effective treatments for tuberculosis). Aminoglycosides enter bacterial cells via an oxygen-dependent transport system. Streptococci and anaerobic bacteria do not have this transport system, so have innate aminoglycoside resistance. Other bacteria acquire resistance through reduced cell membrane permeability to aminoglycosides or acquisition of enzymes that modify aminoglycosides to prevent them from reaching the ribosomes. As penicillins weaken bacterial cell walls, they may enhance aminoglycoside activity by increasing bacterial uptake.
Important adverse effects	The most important adverse effects are **nephrotoxicity** and **ototoxicity.** Aminoglycosides accumulate in renal tubular epithelial cells and cochlear and vestibular hair cells where they trigger apoptosis and cell death. Nephrotoxicity presents as reduced urine output and rising serum creatinine and urea and is potentially reversible. Ototoxicity is often not noticed until after resolution of the acute infection, when the patient may complain of hearing loss, tinnitus (cochlear damage) and/or vertigo (vestibular damage). Ototoxicity may be irreversible.
Warnings	Aminoglycosides are renally excreted. Monitoring of plasma drug concentrations with careful dose adjustment is essential to prevent renal, cochlear and vestibular damage, particularly in ▲**neonates** and the ▲**elderly** who are most susceptible and in patients with ▲**renal impairment.** Aminoglycosides can impair neuromuscular transmission so should not be given to people with ▲**myasthenia gravis** unless absolutely necessary.
Important interactions	**Ototoxicity** is more likely if aminoglycosides are co-prescribed with <u>loop diuretics</u> (e.g. furosemide) or <u>vancomycin</u>. **Nephrotoxicity** is more likely if aminoglycosides are co-prescribed with ciclosporin, platinum chemotherapy, <u>cephalosporins</u> or <u>vancomycin</u>.

PRACTICAL PRESCRIBING

Prescription	Aminoglycosides are highly polarised, so do not cross lipid membranes and therefore **cannot be given orally.** In severe infection, parenteral aminoglycosides (e.g. gentamicin) are usually given as a **once daily IV infusion.** The dose of aminoglycoside is calculated from the patient's weight (see Clinical tip) and renal function. For example, the gentamicin dose may be 5 mg/kg with normal renal function and 3 mg/kg with severe renal impairment. The dose interval (time between doses) is determined by **drug level monitoring,** with subsequent doses being administered only when plasma concentrations have fallen to a safe level (see Monitoring). The dose interval is usually 24 hours for people with normal renal function and longer (e.g. 36–48 hours) in renal impairment. Treatment duration should be as short as possible to limit toxicity, often a single dose and usually less than 7 days.
Administration	For **IV administration,** aminoglycosides should be diluted (e.g. in 50 mL sodium chloride 0.9%) and infused slowly (e.g. over 30 minutes). This prevents exposure of the ear to a high concentration bolus of aminoglycosides (a potential hazard of impatience during IV injection).
Communication	Explain that the aim of treatment is to get rid of infection and improve symptoms. Ask the patient daily if they have noticed any **change in their hearing, ringing in their ears or dizziness** and advise them to let you know if this occurs. Ensure that the prescription clearly indicates that **dosing depends on plasma concentrations** and that measurement and recording of these has been organised, particularly at weekends.
Monitoring	For **efficacy,** monitor symptoms and signs (e.g. pyrexia) and blood inflammatory markers (e.g. C-reactive protein) to ensure resolution of infection. For **safety,** renal function should be measured before (to guide dosing) and during (to detect toxicity) parenteral aminoglycoside therapy. The **plasma drug concentration** is usually measured 18–24 hours after the first dose (trough level). The next dose should only be administered if these have fallen to a safe level with a low risk of toxicity (e.g. gentamicin <1 mg/mL). If the plasma concentration is too high, the next dose should be withheld until repeat levels indicate that it is safe to give.
Cost	Cost is not usually a consideration when prescribing aminoglycosides for life-threatening infection. Short courses are inexpensive.

Clinical tip—In obese patients, aminoglycosides should be dosed according to their ideal weight-for-height (e.g. http://www.calculator.net/ideal-weight-calculator.html; accessed 24/02/2014), rather than their actual body weight, to prevent excessive dosing.

Aminosalicylates

CLINICAL PHARMACOLOGY

Common indications	❶ Mesalazine is used first-line in the treatment of mild-to-moderate **ulcerative colitis;** sulfasalazine is an alternative but has largely been replaced by mesalazine for this indication. ❷ Sulfasalazine is one of several options for the management of **rheumatoid arthritis,** in which it is used as a disease-modifying antirheumatic drug (DMARD), usually as part of combination therapy.
Mechanisms of action	In ulcerative colitis (UC), mesalazine and sulfasalazine both exert their therapeutic effects by releasing **5-aminosalicylic acid (5-ASA).** The precise mechanism of action of 5-ASA is unknown, but it has both **anti-inflammatory and immunosuppressive effects,** and appears to act topically on the gut rather than systemically. For this reason, 5-ASA preparations are designed to delay delivery of the active ingredient to the colon. The oral form of mesalazine comprises a tablet with a coating that resists gastric breakdown, instead releasing 5-ASA further down the gut. Sulfasalazine consists of a molecule of 5-ASA linked to sulfapyridine. In the colon, bacterial enzymes break this link and release the two molecules. Sulfapyridine does not contribute to its therapeutic effect in UC, but it does cause side effects, and for this reason it has largely been replaced by mesalazine for this indication. By contrast, sulfapyridine is probably active in rheumatoid arthritis, though its mechanism is unclear. Mesalazine has no role in rheumatoid arthritis.
Important adverse effects	Mesalazine generally causes fewer side effects than sulfasalazine. Most commonly, these are **gastrointestinal upset** (e.g. nausea, dyspepsia) and **headache.** Both drugs can cause rare but serious blood abnormalities (e.g. **leucopenia, thrombocytopenia**) and **renal impairment.** In men, sulfasalazine may induce a reversible decrease in the number of sperm (**oligospermia**). It can also cause a **serious hypersensitivity reaction** comprising fever, rash and liver abnormalities.
Warnings	Mesalazine and sulfasalazine are salicylates, like aspirin. Patients who have ✖**aspirin hypersensitivity** should not take these drugs.
Important interactions	Mesalazine tablets with a pH-sensitive coating (e.g. Asacol® MR) may interact with drugs that alter gut pH. For example, proton pump inhibitors increase gastric pH so may cause the coating to be broken down prematurely. Lactulose lowers stool pH and may prevent 5-ASA release in the colon.

PRACTICAL PRESCRIBING

Prescription | In patients with rectal or rectosigmoid **ulcerative colitis,** a mesalazine enema or suppository is generally recommended in the first instance. In an acute attack, this is taken once or twice daily for 4–6 weeks in an attempt to induce remission. If the disease is more proximal, or the patient would prefer not to take the drug rectally, an oral formulation may be used. Drug choice (and therefore dosage regimen) is likely to be dictated by local policies. Decisions regarding choice of therapy in **rheumatoid arthritis** should be taken by a specialist.

Administration | The commonly used Asacol® foam enema requires thorough mixing before administration, by shaking the can vigorously for two 15-second periods. An applicator is then attached, and this is inserted as far as possible into the rectum. The can must be upside-down when the dome is pressed and released to deliver a dose. The applicator should then be removed and disposed of cleanly, and the patient should wash their hands. For suppositories, patients should empty their bowels first if necessary, insert the suppository, then avoid opening their bowels for at least an hour if possible. Tablet forms of mesalazine should be swallowed whole; not chewed or crushed.

Communication | Explain the aim of treatment as appropriate for the indication. Ensure the patient understands how to take the medicine, particularly if it is a rectal preparation (see Administration and Clinical tip). Ask them to report any unexplained bleeding, bruising, or infective symptoms to a doctor as soon as possible, since this could be a sign of a blood count abnormality that may require urgent assessment.

Monitoring | The best guide to **efficacy** in ulcerative colitis is the patient's symptoms. In rheumatoid arthritis, this may be supplemented by the C-reactive protein concentration and calculation of disease activity scores. For **safety,** renal function should be checked in patients receiving oral mesalazine, and full blood count and liver profile monitored in patients receiving sulfasalazine.

Cost | Mesalazine is available in a number of branded forms which vary in price. Choice is likely to be dictated by local formulary agreements.

Clinical tip—Administration of the rectal forms of mesalazine is not easy, particularly for patients with active ulcerative colitis. Give patients written advice and ensure they understand this. For those using a foam enema, consider supplying (or advising them to obtain) a water-based lubricant to facilitate insertion of the applicator. Similarly, insertion of suppositories can be made easier by greasing their tip with a little petroleum jelly.

Amiodarone

CLINICAL PHARMACOLOGY

Common indications	❶ In the management of a wide range of **tachyarrhythmias,** including atrial fibrillation (AF), atrial flutter, supraventricular tachycardia (SVT), ventricular tachycardia (VT) and refractory ventricular fibrillation (VF). It is generally used only when other therapeutic options (drugs or electrical cardioversion) are ineffective or inappropriate.
Mechanisms of action	Amiodarone has many effects on myocardial cells, including **blockade of sodium, calcium and potassium channels,** and **antagonism of α- and β-adrenergic receptors.** These effects reduce spontaneous depolarisation (automaticity), slow conduction velocity, and increase resistance to depolarisation (refractoriness), including in the atrioventricular (AV) node. By interfering with AV node conduction, amiodarone reduces the ventricular rate in AF and atrial flutter. Through its other effects, it may also increase the chance of conversion to, and maintenance of, sinus rhythm. In SVT involving a self-perpetuating ('re-entry') circuit that includes the AV node, amiodarone may break the circuit and restore sinus rhythm. Amiodarone's effects in suppressing spontaneous depolarisations make it an option for both treatment and prevention of VT. The same rationale underlies its use in refractory VF, although there is little evidence from clinical trials to support this.
Important adverse effects	In acute use, compared with other antiarrhythmic drugs, amiodarone causes relatively little myocardial depression, although it can cause **hypotension** during IV infusion. When taken chronically, it has many side effects, a number of which are serious. These include effects on the lungs (**pneumonitis**), heart (**bradycardia, AV block**), liver (**hepatitis**) and skin (**photosensitivity** and **grey discolouration**). Due to its iodine content (am/ODarone) and structural similarities to thyroid hormone, it may cause **thyroid abnormalities,** including hypo- and hyperthyroidism. Amiodarone has an extremely long half-life. After discontinuation, it may take months to be completely eliminated.
Warnings	Amiodarone is a potentially dangerous drug that should be used only when the risk–benefit balance justifies this. It should specifically be avoided in patients with ▲**severe hypotension,** ▲**heart block** and ▲**active thyroid disease.**
Important interactions	Amiodarone interacts with many drugs – too many to list here. Notably, it increases plasma concentrations of ▲<u>digoxin</u>, ▲<u>diltiazem</u> and ▲<u>verapamil</u>. This may increase the risk of bradycardia, AV block and heart failure. The doses of these drugs should be halved if amiodarone is started.

PRACTICAL PRESCRIBING

Prescription	A decision to prescribe amiodarone, whether for acute or long-term use, always requires senior involvement and should not be taken independently by a foundation doctor. One exception is in **cardiac arrest,** in which it is given for VF or pulseless VT immediately after the third shock in the Advanced Life Support algorithm. The dose is 300 mg IV, followed by 20 mL of 0.9% sodium chloride or 5% glucose as a flush. In this instance, it should be administered first and prescribed later.
Administration	In cardiac arrest, amiodarone is given as a bolus injection. It is often provided in a pre-filled syringe to facilitate easy administration. It should be given through the 'best' IV cannula available. Outside cardiac arrests, if continuous or repeated IV infusions are anticipated, these should be given via a **central line.** This is because peripheral intravenous administration can cause significant phlebitis.
Communication	As appropriate, explain that you are advising treatment aimed at correcting their fast or irregular heart rhythm. Explain that it has a number of important and potentially serious side effects, and it is being used only because their condition is serious and no other treatments are suitable. In long-term use, ask the patient to report any symptoms of breathlessness, persistent cough, jaundice, restlessness, weight loss, tiredness or weight gain. Advise the patient not to drink grapefruit juice, as this can increase the risk of side effects, and to avoid exposure of their skin to direct sunlight due to the risk of photosensitivity.
Monitoring	The **efficacy** of treatment is best judged by monitoring the patient's heart rate and rhythm. For **safety,** IV infusion should be accompanied by continuous cardiac monitoring. In long-term therapy, baseline tests should include renal, liver and thyroid profiles, and a chest X-ray. The liver and thyroid profiles should then be repeated 6-monthly.
Cost	Amiodarone is cheap; cost is not material to prescribing decisions.

Clinical tip—While foundation doctors should never initiate amiodarone independently, they may need to re-write prescriptions for ongoing therapy. Always confirm whether it is appropriate to continue amiodarone and, if you are in any doubt, consult a senior colleague. When writing the prescription, do not blindly copy the preceding dose. This may have being a **loading dose** (which seeks to achieve therapeutic concentrations rapidly), whereas you probably need to prescribe a **maintenance dose.** Again, never hesitate to seek advice. If you find yourself prescribing amiodarone on a discharge prescription, always confirm with a senior colleague whether this is appropriate. If the acute problems have resolved, it may be possible to stop it.

Angiotensin-converting enzyme (ACE) inhibitors

CLINICAL PHARMACOLOGY

Common indications	❶ **Hypertension:** for the first- or second-line treatment of hypertension, to reduce the risk of stroke, myocardial infarction and death from cardiovascular disease. ❷ **Chronic heart failure:** for the first-line treatment of all grades of heart failure, to improve symptoms and prognosis. ❸ **Ischaemic heart disease:** to reduce the risk of subsequent cardiovascular events such as myocardial infarction and stroke. ❹ **Diabetic nephropathy** and **chronic kidney disease (CKD) with proteinuria:** to reduce proteinuria and progression of nephropathy.
Mechanisms of action	ACE inhibitors block the action of the ACE, to **prevent the conversion of angiotensin I to angiotensin II.** Angiotensin II is a vasoconstrictor and stimulates aldosterone secretion. Blocking its action reduces peripheral vascular resistance (afterload), which lowers blood pressure. It particularly dilates the efferent glomerular arteriole, which reduces intraglomerular pressure and slows the progression of CKD. Reducing the aldosterone level promotes sodium and water excretion. This can help to reduce venous return (preload), which has a beneficial effect in heart failure.
Important adverse effects	Common side effects include **hypotension** (particularly after the **first dose**), **persistent dry cough** (due to increased levels of bradykinin, which is usually inactivated by ACE) and **hyperkalaemia** (because a lower aldosterone level promotes potassium retention). They can cause or worsen **renal failure.** This is particularly relevant in patients with renal artery stenosis, who rely on constriction of the efferent glomerular arteriole to maintain glomerular filtration. If detected early, these adverse effects are usually reversible on stopping the drug. Rare but important idiosyncratic side effects of ACE inhibitors include **angioedema** and other **anaphylactoid reactions.**
Warnings	ACE inhibitors should be avoided in patients with ✖**renal artery stenosis** or ✖**acute kidney injury;** in women who are, or could become, ▲**pregnant;** and those who are ▲**breastfeeding.** Although ACE inhibition is potentially valuable in some forms of ▲**chronic kidney disease,** lower doses should be used and the effect on renal function monitored closely.
Important interactions	Due to the risk of hyperkalaemia, avoid prescribing ACE inhibitors with other ▲**potassium-elevating drugs,** including <u>potassium supplements</u> (<u>oral</u> or <u>IV</u>) and <u>potassium-sparing diuretics</u> except under specialist advice for advanced heart failure. In combination with other diuretics they may be associated with profound first-dose hypotension. The combination of an ▲<u>NSAID</u> and an ACE inhibitor increases the risk of renal failure.

PRACTICAL PRESCRIBING

Prescription	ACE inhibitors are taken orally. The starting dose varies according to the indication, generally being lower in heart failure than in other indications. A common choice is ramipril 1.25 mg daily in heart failure or nephropathy, or 2.5 mg daily in most other indications. This is **'titrated up'** to a maximum 10 mg daily dose over a period of weeks, according to the patient's response, side effects and renal function.
Administration	They can be taken with or without food. It is best to take the **first dose before bed** to reduce symptomatic hypotension.
Communication	Explain that you are offering treatment with a medicine to improve blood pressure and reduce strain on their heart. Advise patients about common side effects such as a **dry cough,** and about the possibility of **dizziness** due to low blood pressure, particularly after the first dose. Mention that, very rarely, this medicine can cause effects similar to severe **allergic reactions;** they should stop taking it and seek urgent medical advice if they develop facial swelling or stomach pains. Make sure they understand the need for **blood test monitoring**, explaining that ACE inhibitors can interfere with their kidney function and upset potassium balance. Advise them to **avoid** taking over-the-counter **anti-inflammatories** (e.g. ibuprofen) due to the risk of kidney damage.
Monitoring	Monitor **efficacy** clinically, for example reduced **symptoms** of breathlessness in heart failure, or improved **blood pressure** control in hypertension. For **safety,** check **electrolytes** and **renal function** before starting treatment. Repeat these 1–2 weeks into treatment and after increasing the dose. Biochemical changes can be tolerated provided they are within certain limits: the creatinine concentration should not rise by more than 30%, the eGFR should not fall by more than 25%, and the potassium concentration should not rise above 6.0 mmol/L. If any of these limits are exceeded, you should stop the drug and seek expert advice.
Cost	Most ACE inhibitors are available as non-proprietary products, which are inexpensive. There is generally no reason to use a branded product, which can be significantly more expensive.

Clinical tip—Profound hypotension may occur following the first dose of an ACE inhibitor, particularly in patients on other diuretics, such as loop diuretics, and those with restricted salt and water intake. You should start at a low dose and titrate up gradually. In addition, it can sometimes be advisable to omit the diuretic dose that precedes the first dose of the ACE inhibitor.

Angiotensin receptor blockers

CLINICAL PHARMACOLOGY

Common indications	Angiotensin receptor blockers (ARBs) are generally used when <u>ACE inhibitors</u> are not tolerated due to cough. The indications are the same: ❶ **Hypertension:** for the first- or second-line treatment of hypertension, to reduce the risk of stroke, myocardial infarction and death from cardiovascular disease. ❷ **Chronic heart failure:** for the first-line treatment of all grades of heart failure, to improve symptoms and prognosis. ❸ **Ischaemic heart disease:** to reduce the risk of subsequent cardiovascular events such as myocardial infarction and stroke. ❹ **Diabetic nephropathy** and **chronic kidney disease (CKD) with proteinuria:** to reduce proteinuria and progression of nephropathy.
Mechanisms of action	ARBs have similar effects to ACE inhibitors, but instead of inhibiting the conversion of angiotensin I to angiotensin II, ARBs **block the action of angiotensin II on the AT_1 receptor.** Angiotensin II is a vasoconstrictor and stimulates aldosterone secretion. Blocking its action reduces peripheral vascular resistance (afterload), which lowers blood pressure. It particularly dilates the efferent glomerular arteriole, which reduces intraglomerular pressure and slows the progression of CKD. Reducing the aldosterone level promotes sodium and water excretion. This can help to reduce venous return (preload), which has a beneficial effect in heart failure.
Important adverse effects	ARBs can cause **hypotension** (particularly after the **first dose**), **hyperkalaemia** and **renal failure.** The mechanism is the same as for ACE inhibitors. Patients most at risk of renal failure are those with renal artery stenosis, who rely on constriction of the efferent glomerular arteriole to maintain glomerular filtration. Unlike ACE inhibitors, ARBs are less likely to cause a dry cough, as they do not inhibit ACE, and therefore do not affect bradykinin metabolism. For the same reason, they are less likely to cause angioedema.
Warnings	ARBs should be avoided in patients with ✖**renal artery stenosis** or ✖**acute kidney injury;** in women who are, or could become, ▲**pregnant;** and those who are ▲**breastfeeding.** Although ARB therapy is potentially valuable in some forms of ▲**chronic kidney disease,** lower doses should be used and the effect on renal function monitored closely.
Important interactions	Due to the risk of hyperkalaemia, avoid prescribing ARBs with other ▲**potassium-elevating drugs,** including <u>potassium supplements</u> (<u>oral</u> or <u>IV</u>) and <u>potassium-sparing diuretics</u> except under specialist advice for advanced heart failure. In combination with other diuretics they may be associated with profound first-dose hypotension. The combination of <u>NSAIDs</u> with ARBs increases the risk of renal failure.

PRACTICAL PRESCRIBING

Prescription	ARBs are taken **orally.** The starting dose varies according to the indication, generally being lower in heart failure than in other indications. A common choice is losartan 12.5 mg daily in heart failure or 50 mg daily in other indications. This is '**titrated up**' to the maximum recommended dose over a period of weeks, according to the patient's response, side effects and renal function.
Administration	They can be taken with or without food. It is best to take **the first dose before bed** to reduce symptomatic hypotension.
Communication	Explain that you are offering treatment with a medicine to improve their blood pressure and reduce strain on their heart. If the patient has previously been unable to tolerate an ACE inhibitor due to cough, explain that the new treatment does not cause this side effect. Advise patients about the possibility of **dizziness** due to low blood pressure, particularly after the first dose. Make sure they understand the need for **blood test monitoring,** explaining that ARBs can interfere with their kidney function and upset potassium balance. Advise them to **avoid taking** over-the-counter anti-inflammatories (e.g. ibuprofen) due to the risk of kidney damage.
Monitoring	Monitor **efficacy** clinically, for example reduced **symptoms** of breathlessness in heart failure, or improved **blood pressure** control in hypertension. For **safety,** check **electrolytes** and **renal function** before starting treatment. Repeat this 1–2 weeks into treatment and after increasing the dose. Biochemical changes can be tolerated provided they are within certain limits: the creatinine concentration should not rise by more than 30%, the eGFR should not fall by more than 25%, and the potassium concentration should not rise above 6.0 mmol/L. If any of these limits are exceeded, you should stop the drug and seek expert advice.
Cost	Losartan is available in non-proprietary form and is inexpensive; the equivalent brand name form costs about two times more. There is no compelling reason to choose a branded product over a non-proprietary one.

Clinical tip—The incidence of angioedema related to ACE inhibitor treatment is five times higher (about 1%) in black people of African or Caribbean origin. The exact mechanism by which ACE inhibitors lead to angioedema is not completely understood but is thought to relate to altered bradykinin metabolism. ARBs do not affect levels of bradykinin and are less likely to cause angioedema. They therefore may be preferable to ACE inhibitors in this group.

Antidepressants, selective serotonin reuptake inhibitors

CLINICAL PHARMACOLOGY

Common indications	**❶** As first-line treatment for **moderate-to-severe depression,** and in **mild depression** if psychological treatments fail. **❷ Panic disorder.** **❸ Obsessive compulsive disorder.**
Mechanisms of action	Selective serotonin reuptake inhibitors (SSRIs) preferentially **inhibit neuronal reuptake of serotonin** (5-HT) from the synaptic cleft, thereby increasing its availability for neurotransmission. This appears to be the mechanism by which SSRIs improve mood and physical symptoms in depression and relieve symptoms of panic and obsessive disorders. SSRIs differ from <u>tricyclic antidepressants</u> in that they do not inhibit noradrenaline uptake and cause less blockade of other receptors. The efficacy of the two drug classes in the treatment of depression is similar. However, SSRIs are generally preferred as they have fewer adverse effects and are less dangerous in overdose.
Important adverse effects	Common adverse effects include **gastrointestinal upset, appetite and weight disturbance** (loss or gain) and **hypersensitivity** reactions, including skin rash. **Hyponatraemia** is an important adverse effect, particularly in the elderly, and may present with confusion and reduced consciousness. **Suicidal thoughts and behaviour** may be increased in patients on SSRIs. SSRIs **lower the seizure threshold** and some (e.g. citalopram) **prolong the QT interval** and can predispose to arrhythmias. SSRIs also increase the risk of **bleeding.** At high doses, in overdose, or in combination with other antidepressant classes, SSRIs can cause **serotonin syndrome.** This is a triad of autonomic hyperactivity, altered mental state and neuromuscular excitation, which usually responds to treatment withdrawal and supportive therapy. **Sudden withdrawal** of SSRIs can cause gastrointestinal upset, neurological and influenza-like symptoms and sleep disturbance.
Warnings	SSRIs should be prescribed with caution where there is a particular risk of adverse effects, including in ▲**epilepsy** and ▲**peptic ulcer disease.** In ▲**young people,** SSRIs have poor efficacy and are associated with an increased risk of self-harm and suicidal thoughts, so should only be prescribed by specialists. As SSRIs are metabolised by the liver, dose reduction may be required in people with ▲**hepatic impairment.**
Important interactions	SSRIs should not be given with ✖**monoamine oxidase inhibitors** as they both increase synaptic serotonin levels and together may precipitate serotonin syndrome. Gastroprotection should be prescribed for patients taking SSRIs with <u>aspirin</u> or <u>NSAIDs</u> due to an increased risk of gastrointestinal bleeding. Bleeding risk is also increased where SSRIs are co-prescribed with <u>anticoagulants</u>. They should not be combined with other ▲**drugs that prolong the QT interval,** such as <u>antipsychotics</u>.

citalopram, fluoxetine, sertraline, escitalopram

PRACTICAL PRESCRIBING

Prescription	SSRIs are only available for oral administration. They should be started at a low dose to be taken regularly, usually once a day. A typical starting prescription might be for citalopram 20 mg orally daily. The dose is increased as necessary according to response. Lower starting and maximum doses are prescribed for elderly patients.
Administration	Citalopram is available as tablets and as oral drops, which can be mixed with water or other drinks. As the oral drops have greater bioavailability than tablets, they are prescribed at different doses. For example, one 20 mg citalopram tablet is equivalent to 16 mg citalopram in 4 oral drops.
Communication	Advise patients that treatment should **improve symptoms** over a few weeks, particularly sleep and appetite. Discuss referring them for **psychological therapy,** which may offer more long-term benefits than drug treatment. Explain that they should carry on with drug treatment for **at least 6 months** after they feel better to stop the depression from coming back (2 years for recurrent depression). Warn them **not to stop treatment suddenly** as this may cause a tummy upset, flu-like **withdrawal symptoms** and sleeplessness. When the time comes to stop treatment, they should reduce the dose slowly over 4 weeks. While patients may find some of the more common side effects unpleasant, they may tolerate them in favour of relieving depressive symptoms. Discussing at an early stage what side effects are expected may encourage patients to persist with treatment; at least until the full antidepressant effects are realised.
Monitoring	Symptoms should be reviewed 1–2 weeks after starting treatment and regularly thereafter. If no effect has been seen at 4 weeks, you should consider changing the dose or drug. Otherwise the dose should not be adjusted until after 6–8 weeks of therapy.
Cost	Most SSRIs are available in non-proprietary form and are inexpensive.

Clinical tip—Citalopram and escitalopram appear to have fewer interactions than other SSRIs. You should therefore consider choosing these drugs when prescribing antidepressants for patients with multiple comorbidities who are taking lots of other drugs.

Antidepressants, tricyclics and related drugs

CLINICAL PHARMACOLOGY

Common indications	❶ As second-line treatment for **moderate-to-severe depression** where first-line <u>serotonin-specific reuptake inhibitors</u> (SSRIs) are ineffective. ❷ As a treatment option for **neuropathic pain,** although they are not licensed for this indication.
Mechanisms of action	Tricyclic antidepressants **inhibit neuronal reuptake of serotonin (5-HT) and noradrenaline** from the synaptic cleft, thereby increasing their availability for neurotransmission. This appears to be the mechanism by which they improve mood and physical symptoms in moderate-to-severe (but not mild) depression and probably accounts for their effect in modifying neuropathic pain. 　Tricyclic antidepressants also **block a wide array of receptors,** including muscarinic, histamine (H_1), α-adrenergic (α_1 and α_2) and dopamine (D_2) receptors. This accounts for the extensive adverse effects profile that limits their clinical utility.
Important adverse effects	Blockade of **antimuscarinic** receptors causes dry mouth, constipation, urinary retention and blurred vision. Blockade of H_1 and α_1 receptors causes **sedation** and **hypotension.** Cardiac adverse effects (multiple mechanisms) include **arrhythmias** and **ECG changes** (including prolongation of the QT and QRS durations). In the brain, more serious effects include **convulsions, hallucinations** and **mania.** Blockade of dopamine receptors can cause **breast changes** and **sexual dysfunction** and rarely causes **extrapyramidal symptoms** (tremor and dyskinesia). Tricyclic antidepressants are extremely **dangerous in overdose,** causing severe hypotension, arrhythmias, convulsions, coma and respiratory failure, which can be fatal. 　**Sudden withdrawal** of tricyclic antidepressants can cause gastrointestinal upset, neurological and influenza-like symptoms and sleep disturbance.
Warnings	Tricyclic antidepressants should be used with caution in people who are particularly at risk of adverse effects. These include the ▲**elderly,** people with ▲**cardiovascular disease** or ▲**epilepsy**, and people with ▲**constipation,** ▲**prostatic hypertrophy** or ▲**raised intraocular pressure,** which may be worsened by antimuscarinic effects.
Important interactions	Tricyclic antidepressants should not be given with ✖**monoamine oxidase inhibitors** as both drug classes increase serotonin and noradrenaline levels at the synapse and together they can precipitate hypertension and hyperthermia or serotonin syndrome (see <u>Antidepressants, selective serotonin reuptake inhibitors</u>). Tricyclic antidepressants can augment antimuscarinic, sedative or hypotensive adverse effects of other drugs.

PRACTICAL PRESCRIBING

Prescription	**Depression:** Tricyclic antidepressants have similar efficacy to other classes of antidepressant (e.g. SSRIs), but have more adverse effects and are more dangerous in overdose. They are therefore reserved for patients in whom SSRIs are ineffective and should only be prescribed by a healthcare professional with relevant mental health training. For depression, tricyclic antidepressants with fewer adverse effects are preferred, e.g. lofepramine. **Neuropathic pain:** Amitriptyline is used at a much lower dose (e.g. starting dose 10 mg at night) for this indication than for depression (where starting dose is 75 mg daily).
Administration	Tricyclic antidepressants are available as tablets and in oral solution. When prescribing for depression, particularly for people who are at risk of suicide, it is good practice to **supply a small quantity** of medication at a time (e.g. enough for 2 weeks) to reduce the risk of serious overdose.
Communication	Advise patients that treatment will **improve symptoms** over a few weeks, particularly sleep and appetite. Discuss referring them for **psychological therapy,** which may offer more long-term benefits than drug treatment. Explain that they should carry on with drug treatment for **at least 6 months** after they feel better to stop the depression from coming back (2 years for recurrent depression). Warn them **not to stop treatment suddenly** as this may cause flu-like **withdrawal symptoms** and sleeplessness. When the time comes to stop treatment, they should reduce the dose slowly over 4 weeks. While patients may find some of the more common side effects unpleasant, they may tolerate them in favour of relieving depressive symptoms. Discussing at an early stage what side effects are expected may encourage patients to persist with treatment; at least until the full antidepressant effects are realised.
Monitoring	Symptoms should be reviewed 1–2 weeks after starting treatment and regularly thereafter. If no effect has been seen at 4 weeks, you should consider changing the dose or drug. Otherwise the dose should not be adjusted until after 6–8 weeks of therapy.
Cost	Tricyclic antidepressants are available as non-proprietary preparations and are inexpensive.

Clinical tip—It was previously thought to take 2–4 weeks for antidepressant therapy to take effect. However, it has now been demonstrated that relief of symptoms develops and evolves from the first week in therapy.

Antidepressants, venlafaxine and mirtazapine

CLINICAL PHARMACOLOGY

Common indications	❶ As an option for treatment of **major depression** where first-line selective serotonin reuptake inhibitors (SSRIs) are ineffective or not tolerated. ❷ **Generalised anxiety disorder** (venlafaxine).
Mechanisms of action	*Venlafaxine* is a serotonin and noradrenaline reuptake inhibitor (SNRI), interfering with uptake of these neurotransmitters from the synaptic cleft. *Mirtazapine* is an antagonist of inhibitory pre-synaptic α_2-adrenoceptors. **Both drugs increase availability of monoamines for neurotransmission,** which appears to be the mechanism whereby they improve mood and physical symptoms in moderate-to-severe (but not mild) depression. Venlafaxine is a weaker antagonist of muscarinic and histamine (H_1) receptors than tricyclic antidepressants, whereas mirtazapine is a potent antagonist of histamine (H_1) but not muscarinic receptors. They therefore have fewer antimuscarinic side effects than tricyclic antidepressants, although mirtazapine commonly causes sedation.
Important adverse effects	Common adverse effects of both drugs include **gastrointestinal upset** (e.g. dry mouth, nausea, change in weight and diarrhoea or constipation) and **central nervous system effects** (e.g. headache, abnormal dreams, insomnia, confusion and convulsions). Less common but serious adverse effects include **hyponatraemia** and **serotonin syndrome** (see Antidepressants, selective serotonin reuptake inhibitors). **Suicidal thoughts and behaviour** may increase. Venlafaxine prolongs the QT interval and can increase the risk of ventricular arrhythmias. **Sudden drug withdrawal** can cause gastrointestinal upset, neurological and influenza-like symptoms and sleep disturbance. Venlafaxine is associated with a greater risk of withdrawal effects than other antidepressants.
Warnings	As with many centrally acting medications, the ▲elderly are at particular risk of adverse effects. A dose reduction should be considered in people with ▲hepatic or ▲renal impairment. Venlafaxine should be used with caution (if at all) in patients with ▲cardiovascular disease associated with an increased risk of arrhythmias.
Important interactions	The combination of these drugs with drugs from other antidepressant classes can increase the risk of adverse effects (including serotonin syndrome, see Antidepressants, selective serotonin reuptake inhibitors) and should, in general, be avoided.

PRACTICAL PRESCRIBING

Prescription	Venlafaxine and mirtazapine are only available for oral administration. They should usually be prescribed by a healthcare professional with relevant mental health training and used in conjunction with psychological therapies. As with other antidepressants, treatment is started at a low dose and titrated up according to response. Typical starting doses are venlafaxine 37.5 mg orally twice daily (titrated to a maximum of 375 mg daily) and mirtazapine 15 mg orally daily (titrated to a maximum of 45 mg daily).
Administration	Mirtazapine should be taken at night to minimise (or benefit from!) its sedative effects.
Communication	Advise patients that treatment should **improve symptoms** over a few weeks, particularly sleep and appetite. Discuss referring them for **psychological therapy,** which may offer more long-term benefits than drug treatment. Explain that they should carry on with drug treatment for **at least 6 months** after they feel better to stop the depression from coming back (2 years for recurrent depression). Warn them **not to stop treatment suddenly** as this may cause flu-like **withdrawal symptoms** and sleeplessness. When the time comes to stop treatment, they should reduce the dose slowly over 4 weeks. Warn patients taking *mirtazapine* to seek medical advice for symptoms of infection, such as sore throat, so that a blood test can be taken to check for blood disorders. While patients may find some of the more common side effects unpleasant, they may tolerate them in favour of relieving depressive symptoms. Discussing at an early stage what side effects are expected may encourage patients to persist with treatment; at least until the full antidepressant effects are realised.
Monitoring	Symptoms should be reviewed 1–2 weeks after starting treatment and regularly thereafter. If no effect has been seen at 4 weeks, you should consider changing the dose or drug. Otherwise the dose should not be adjusted until after 6–8 weeks of therapy.
Cost	Both drugs are available in non-proprietary form and are relatively inexpensive.

Clinical tip—Perhaps counterintuitively, there is some evidence to suggest that the sedative effects of mirtazapine are *less severe* at *higher* doses than at lower doses. In theory, this may be because at low dose the antihistamine effects of mirtazapine predominate. By contrast, at higher doses, augmented monoamine transmission counteracts the sedating effects of H_1 receptor antagonism. However, as it is not proven that this phenomenon occurs at clinical doses (15–45 mg), we would not advocate routinely increasing the dose of mirtazapine to overcome sedation or somnolence.

Antiemetics, dopamine D₂-receptor antagonists

CLINICAL PHARMACOLOGY

Common indications	❶ Prophylaxis and treatment of **nausea and vomiting** in a wide range of conditions, but particularly in the context of **reduced gut motility.**
Mechanisms of action	Nausea and vomiting are triggered by a variety of factors, including gut irritation, drugs, motion and vestibular disorders, as well as higher stimuli (sights, smells, emotions). The various pathways converge on a 'vomiting centre' in the medulla, which receives inputs from the chemoreceptor trigger zone, the solitary tract nucleus (which is innervated by the vagus nerve), the vestibular system and higher neurological centres. Dopamine, acting via D₂ receptors, is relevant in two respects. First, **the D₂ receptor is the main receptor in the chemoreceptor trigger zone** (CTZ), which is the area responsible for sensing emetogenic substances in the blood (e.g. drugs). Second, dopamine is an important neurotransmitter in the gut, where it promotes relaxation of the stomach and lower oesophageal sphincter and inhibits gastroduodenal coordination. Drugs that block D₂ receptors therefore have a **prokinetic effect** – promoting gastric emptying – which contributes to their antiemetic action. They are effective in nausea and vomiting due to CTZ stimulation (e.g. due to drugs) and reduced gut motility (e.g. due to opioids or diabetic gastroparesis).
Important adverse effects	**Diarrhoea** is probably the most common side effect of D₂-blocking antiemetics. Metoclopramide can induce **extrapyramidal syndromes** (movement abnormalities) via the same mechanism as for antipsychotics. In the context of short-term treatment for nausea and vomiting, this is most likely to take the form of an **acute dystonic reaction** such as an oculogyric crisis. Domperidone tends not to cause extrapyramidal symptoms because it does not cross the blood–brain barrier (note that the chemoreceptor trigger zone is largely outside the blood–brain barrier, so this characteristic does not affect its antiemetic action).
Warnings	Extrapyramidal side effects are more common in ▲**children** and ▲**young adults** so its use should be avoided in these groups. As both drugs have prokinetic effects, they are contraindicated in patients with ▲**gastrointestinal obstruction** and ✖**perforation**.
Important interactions	The risk of extrapyramidal side effects is increased when metoclopramide is prescribed with ▲antipsychotics. It should not be combined with ✖dopaminergic agents for Parkinson's disease, as it will antagonise their effects. Domperidone is not subject to these interactions.

metoclopramide, domperidone

PRACTICAL PRESCRIBING

Prescription	The starting dose for both metoclopramide and domperidone is the same at 10 mg, up to three times daily. Metoclopramide is available for injection (IM/IV); no dosage adjustment is required when switching between routes. Domperidone is not available in an injectable form, although it may be given rectally at a higher dose of 60 mg twice daily. The route of administration, and whether it is prescribed on a regular or as-required basis, depends on the clinical situation. For example, the oral route is clearly inappropriate for a patient who is actively vomiting.
Administration	Intravenous injections of metoclopramide should be given slowly over about 2 minutes for a standard 10 mg dose; by infusion for higher doses.
Communication	Explain that you are offering an anti-sickness medicine. Most people are able to take it without any significant side effects. If you are prescribing outside hospital, it is prudent to mention the possibility of muscle spasms and abnormal movements with metoclopramide. Ask your patient to stop taking the medicine and seek medical attention if they notice any side effects of this type.
Monitoring	Resolution of symptoms is the best guide to efficacy. In prolonged use you should monitor the patient for extrapyramidal features, as these may be subtle (e.g. an increased tendency to falls) and their relationship to the drug may not be obvious to patients or other healthcare professionals.
Cost	Non-proprietary preparations of these drugs are inexpensive. The rectal form of domperidone is relatively more expensive (about 60p per 60 mg dose, compared to as little as 1p per 10 mg oral tablet).

Clinical tip—For patients with gastro-oesophageal reflux disease that does not respond to conventional treatment with a proton pump inhibitor and/or an H_2-receptor antagonist, metoclopramide can be considered as an add-on treatment. Its effects on the lower oesophageal sphincter and gastric emptying may improve the patient's symptoms. Appropriate investigations should have been undertaken to identify treatable causes for reflux symptoms, such as ulcers, *Helicobacter pylori* infection, drugs and cancer.

Antiemetics, histamine H₁-receptor antagonists

CLINICAL PHARMACOLOGY

Common indications	❶ Prophylaxis and treatment of **nausea and vomiting,** particularly in the context of **motion sickness** or **vertigo.**
Mechanisms of action	Nausea and vomiting are triggered by a variety of factors, including gut irritation, drugs, motion and vestibular disorders, as well as higher stimuli (sights, smells, emotions). The various pathways converge on a 'vomiting centre' in the medulla, which receives inputs from the chemoreceptor trigger zone (CTZ), the solitary tract nucleus (which is innervated by the vagus nerve), the vestibular system and higher neurological centres. Histamine (H₁) and acetylcholine (muscarinic) receptors predominate in the **vomiting centre** and in its communication with the **vestibular system.** Drugs such as cyclizine block both of these receptors. This makes them useful treatments for nausea and vomiting in a wide range of conditions (e.g. drug-induced, post-operative, radiotherapy), but most particularly when associated with motion or vertigo.
Important adverse effects	The most common adverse effect is **drowsiness.** Cyclizine is the least sedating drug in this class and is therefore usually preferred. Due to their anticholinergic effects they may cause **dry throat and mouth.** This is usually undesirable, but in patients with copious mucosal secretions it may be beneficial. After IV injection they may cause transient **tachycardia,** which the patient may notice as **palpitations.** Along with their central anticholinergic effects (excitation or depression) this may make for a rather unpleasant experience.
Warnings	Due to their sedating effect, these drugs should be avoided in patients at risk of ▲**hepatic encephalopathy.** They should also be avoided in patients susceptible to anticholinergic side effects, such as those with ▲**prostatic hypertrophy** (who may develop urinary retention).
Important interactions	Sedation may be greater when combined with other sedative drugs (e.g. benzodiazepines, opioids). Anticholinergic effects may be more pronounced in patients taking ipratropium or tiotropium.

cyclizine, cinnarizine, promethazine

PRACTICAL PRESCRIBING

Prescription	A typical prescription might be for cyclizine 50 mg 8-hrly as required. It may be given orally, IV or IM; no dosage adjustment is required when switching between routes. The route of administration, and whether it is prescribed on a regular or as-required basis, depends on the clinical situation. For example, the oral route is clearly inappropriate for a patient who is actively vomiting. As IM injections are painful and rapid IV injections are unpleasant (see Adverse effects), we would suggest that *slow* IV injection is the best choice when oral administration is inappropriate.
Administration	Intravenous injections of cyclizine should be given slowly (over about 2 minutes).
Communication	Explain that you are offering an anti-sickness medicine. Although it is generally effective, it does not work for everyone and a second or different medicine may be necessary. Ask them to let you know if they do not achieve satisfactory relief. Advise that it may cause drowsiness and impair the ability to perform tasks such as driving, which they should therefore avoid.
Monitoring	Resolution of symptoms is the best guide to efficacy.
Cost	The antihistamine antiemetics are relatively inexpensive.

Clinical tip—It is worth noting that hyoscine hydrobromide (an <u>antimuscarinic</u> drug) is an alternative and effective treatment for motion sickness. It is widely used as an over-the-counter remedy for this indication and is effective.

Antiemetics, phenothiazines

CLINICAL PHARMACOLOGY

Common indications	❶ Prophylaxis and treatment of **nausea and vomiting** in a wide range of conditions, particularly when due to **vertigo.** However, due to their side effect profile, <u>other antiemetic classes</u> are usually preferable. ❷ **Psychotic disorders,** such as schizophrenia, where they are used as <u>first-generation (typical) antipsychotics</u>.
Mechanisms of action	Nausea and vomiting are triggered by a variety of factors, including gut irritation, drugs, motion and vestibular disorders, as well as higher stimuli (sights, smells, emotions). The various pathways converge on a 'vomiting centre' in the medulla, which receives inputs from the chemoreceptor trigger zone (CTZ), the solitary tract nucleus (which is innervated by the vagus nerve), the vestibular system and higher neurological centres. The antiemetic properties of phenothiazines arise from blockade of various receptors, including dopamine (D_2) receptors in the CTZ and gut (see <u>Antiemetics, dopamine D_2-receptor antagonists</u>) and, to a lesser extent, histamine (H_1) and acetylcholine (muscarinic) receptors in the **vomiting centre** and **vestibular system** (see <u>Antiemetics, histamine H_1-receptor antagonists</u>). This makes them effective for nausea and vomiting in a wide range of situations, including chemotherapy, radiotherapy and vertigo.
Important adverse effects	**Drowsiness** and **postural hypotension** are relatively common with phenothiazines. Movement abnormalities, termed **extrapyramidal syndromes,** are a major drawback of their use. They arise from D_2 receptor blockade via the same mechanism as for other <u>first-generation (typical) antipsychotics</u>. In the context of short-term treatment for nausea and vomiting, this is most likely to take the form of an **acute dystonic reaction** such as oculogyric crisis. In longer-term treatment (which is more likely when they are used as an antipsychotic), other extrapyramidal syndromes such as **tardive dyskinesia** may occur (see <u>Antipsychotics, first-generation [typical]</u>). Like all antipsychotics, phenothiazines can cause **QT-interval prolongation.**
Warnings	Due to their sedative effect and potential for hepatotoxicity, these drugs should be avoided in patients with ✖**severe liver disease.** They should also be avoided in patients susceptible to anticholinergic side effects, such as those with ▲**prostatic hypertrophy** (who may develop urinary retention). Doses should be reduced in the ▲**elderly.**
Important interactions	You should consult the BNF when prescribing for a patient taking these drugs as there is an extensive list of interactions. Prominent among these are ▲**drugs that prolong the QT interval,** such as <u>antipsychotics</u>, <u>amiodarone</u>, <u>ciprofloxacin</u>, <u>macrolides</u>, <u>quinine</u> and <u>SSRIs.</u>

prochlorperazine, chlorpromazine

PRACTICAL PRESCRIBING

Prescription	We would suggest you seek senior or specialist advice when contemplating prescription of a phenothiazine, as other drugs should usually be tried first. A typical prescription in the context of nausea and vomiting might be for prochlorperazine 20 mg orally or 12.5 mg IM to settle the acute attack, with further oral doses (e.g. 10 mg 12-hrly) prescribed if necessary for ongoing symptoms.
Administration	Intramuscular prochlorperazine should be administered by deep injection in a large muscle.
Communication	Explain that you are offering an anti-sickness medicine. Although it is generally effective, it does not work for everyone and a second or different medicine may be necessary. Ask them to let you know if they do not achieve satisfactory relief. Discuss the potential for drowsiness (and its implications for driving) and dizziness on standing. Ask them to stop taking the medicine and seek medical advice if they develop any muscle spasms or movement abnormalities.
Monitoring	Resolution of symptoms is the best guide to efficacy. In prolonged use you should monitor the patient for extrapyramidal features, as these may be subtle (e.g. an increased tendency to falls) and their relationship to the drug may not be obvious to patients or other healthcare professionals.
Cost	Prochlorperazine is available in inexpensive non-proprietary preparations for oral and IM administration. A buccal tablet is also available; this is a branded product which is about ten times as expensive as the oral form.

Clinical tip—Phenothiazines are not commonly used as a first-line antiemetic in the hospital setting. However, haloperidol (also a first-generation (typical) antipsychotic) is used quite commonly, particularly for opioid-induced nausea. At the low doses required for nausea and vomiting (e.g. 1.5 mg at night) it causes few side effects.

Antiemetics, serotonin 5-HT₃-receptor antagonists

CLINICAL PHARMACOLOGY

Common indications	❶ Prophylaxis and treatment of **nausea and vomiting,** particularly in the context of general anaesthesia and chemotherapy.
Mechanisms of action	Nausea and vomiting are triggered by a variety of factors, including gut irritation, drugs, motion and vestibular disorders, as well as higher stimuli (sights, smells, emotions). The various pathways converge on a 'vomiting centre' in the medulla, which receives inputs from the chemoreceptor trigger zone (CTZ), the solitary tract nucleus (which is innervated by the vagus nerve), the vestibular system and higher neurological centres. Serotonin (5-hydroxytryptamine, 5-HT) plays an important role in two of these pathways. First, **there is a high density of 5-HT₃ receptors in the CTZ,** which are responsible for sensing emetogenic substances in the blood (e.g. drugs). Second, **serotonin is the key neurotransmitter released by the gut** in response to emetogenic stimuli. Acting on 5-HT₃ receptors, it stimulates the vagus nerve, which in turn activates the vomiting centre via the solitary tract nucleus. Of note, serotonin is not involved in communication between the vestibular system and the vomiting centre. Thus 5-HT₃ antagonists are effective against nausea and vomiting due to CTZ stimulation (e.g. drugs) and visceral stimuli (gut infection, radiotherapy), but not in motion sickness.
Important adverse effects	Adverse effects are rare with these medications, although constipation, diarrhoea and headaches can occur.
Warnings	There is a small risk that 5-HT₃ antagonists may prolong the QT interval, although this is usually evident only at high doses (e.g. >16 mg ondansetron). Nevertheless, they should be avoided in patients with a ▲**prolonged QT interval.** If in doubt, review an ECG before prescribing.
Important interactions	Avoid 5-HT₃ antagonists when patients are taking ▲**drugs that prolong the QT interval,** such as antipsychotics, quinine and selective serotonin reuptake inhibitors. If in doubt, check the BNF.

ondansetron, granisetron

PRACTICAL PRESCRIBING

Prescription
A typical starting dose for ondansetron is 4–8 mg 12-hrly, orally or IV. The dosing regimens differ for each indication, with higher doses generally reserved for chemotherapy-induced nausea and vomiting. Oral, rectal and injectable preparations are available. The route of administration, and whether it is prescribed on a regular or as-required basis, depends on the clinical indication. As IM injections are painful, the IV route is usually preferable if oral/rectal administration is inappropriate. Where drugs are used to prevent nausea (e.g. before an anaesthetic), oral doses should be taken an hour before symptoms are anticipated. Intravenous doses can be given immediately before the treatment or procedure.

Administration
There are no special considerations in relation to administration.

Communication
Explain that you are offering an anti-sickness medicine. This is unlikely to cause any significant side effects. Although it is generally effective, it does not work for everyone and a second or different medicine may be necessary. Ask them to let you know if they do not achieve satisfactory relief.

Monitoring
Resolution of symptoms is the best guide to efficacy.

Cost
While non-proprietary formulations exist, 5-HT$_3$ antagonists are still relatively expensive drugs.

Clinical tip—Morning sickness is an unpleasant manifestation of early pregnancy that can be severe enough to require hospitalisation. It can be difficult to treat as drugs administered during the first trimester of pregnancy may cause spontaneous abortion and fetal abnormalities. Although ondansetron is not licensed for morning sickness, a recent historical study of 608,385 women in Denmark found no evidence of adverse fetal outcomes related to taking ondansetron in pregnancy. Ondansetron may therefore be an option for severe morning sickness (e.g. hyperemesis gravidarum) where the benefits outweigh potential risks.

Antifungal drugs

CLINICAL PHARMACOLOGY

Common indications	❶ Treatment of **local fungal infections,** including of the oropharynx, vagina or skin. They may be applied topically (nystatin, clotrimazole) or taken orally (fluconazole). ❷ Systemic treatment of **invasive or disseminated fungal infections.** Specialist treatment is required for these infections, which will not be discussed further in this book.
Mechanisms of action	Fungal cell membranes contain ergosterol. As ergosterol is not seen in animal or human cells it is a target for antifungal drugs. **Polyene antifungals** (e.g. *nystatin*) bind to ergosterol in fungal cell membranes, creating a polar pore which allows intracellular ions to leak out of the cell. This can kill or slow growth of the fungi. **Imidazole** (e.g. *clotrimazole*) and **triazole antifungals** (e.g. *fluconazole*) inhibit ergosterol synthesis, impairing cell membrane synthesis, cell growth and replication. Resistance to antifungals is unusual but can occur during long-term treatment in immunosuppressed patients. Mechanisms include alteration of membrane synthesis to exclude ergosterol, changes in target enzymes or increased drug efflux.
Important adverse effects	Topical *nystatin* and *clotrimazole* have few adverse effects apart from occasional **local irritation** where applied. 　The most common adverse effects of *fluconazole* are **gastrointestinal upset** (including nausea, vomiting, diarrhoea and abdominal pain), **headache, hepatitis** and **hypersensitivity** causing skin rash. Rare but potentially life-threatening reactions include: **severe hepatic toxicity; prolonged QT interval** predisposing to **arrhythmias;** and severe hypersensitivity, including **cutaneous reactions** and **anaphylaxis.**
Warnings	*Nystatin* and *clotrimazole* have no major contraindications. 　*Fluconazole* should be prescribed with caution in patients with ▲**liver disease** because of the risk of hepatic toxicity. A dose reduction is required in ▲**moderate renal impairment.** It should be avoided in ✖**pregnancy** due to the risk of fetal malformation.
Important interactions	There are no significant drug interactions with *nystatin* or *clotrimazole*. 　*Fluconazole* inhibits cytochrome P450 enzymes, causing an increase in plasma concentrations and risk of adverse effects when prescribed with ▲**drugs that are metabolised by P450 enzymes,** including phenytoin, carbamazepine, warfarin, diazepam, simvastatin and sulphonylureas. It may reduce the antiplatelet actions of clopidogrel, a pro-drug which requires activation by liver metabolism. It also increases the risk of serious arrhythmias if prescribed with ▲**drugs that prolong the QT interval,** such as amiodarone, antipsychotics, quinine, quinolone and macrolide antibiotics and SSRIs

PRACTICAL PRESCRIBING

Prescription	*Nystatin* is administered topically as an oral suspension for **oropharyngeal candidiasis** (thrush) at a dose of 100,000 units four times daily for 7 days or until 48 hours after lesions have resolved. It is administered as a cream for **skin infections** at a dose of 100,000 units two to three times daily until 7 days after dermatological lesions have resolved.
	Clotrimazole is used to treat fungal infections of the skin and genital tract, such as **tinea** (ringworm, including athlete's foot) and **candida** (thrush). For skin or mucosal infections, clotrimazole 1% cream (contains 1 g clotrimazole in 100 g cream) is applied two to three times daily until 1–2 weeks after infection has resolved. Clotrimazole is also formulated as a pessary for vaginal candidiasis.
	Oral *fluconazole* is prescribed as a single dose of 150 mg for **vaginal candidiasis.** For **other mucosal infections,** e.g. of the oropharynx, oesophagus and airways, it is prescribed at 50 mg daily for a more prolonged course (e.g. 1–2 weeks). Treatment duration may be longer for **fungal skin infections.** Fluconazole is also available as an intravenous preparation for invasive or disseminated fungal infection.
Administration	Oral *nystatin* should be administered after food and held in the mouth to allow good contact with the lesions. If the patient wears dentures, they should remove them to expose affected areas to treatment.
Communication	Advise patients that, with correct application, treatment should improve symptoms. For skin infections, encourage them to continue treatment for 1–2 weeks after symptoms resolve. Warn patients treated with a prolonged course of *fluconazole* to seek medical advice if they experience any unusual symptoms such as nausea, loss of appetite, lethargy or dark urine which could indicate liver poisoning.
Monitoring	Efficacy can be monitored clinically. For *fluconazole*, liver enzymes should be measured before and during prolonged courses of treatment, particularly where high doses are used, to monitor for hepatic toxicity.
Cost	Nystatin, clotrimazole and fluconazole are inexpensive.

Clinical tip—Elderly hospital inpatients are particularly susceptible to oral candida infection. They are commonly treated with antibiotics and systemic or inhaled corticosteroids, which predispose to oral candidiasis, and with antimuscarinic drugs that reduce saliva (natural defence mechanism). A sore mouth can reduce appetite and delay recovery. Take a torch on your ward round to check for oral candida infection. Encourage mouth care and prescribe nystatin to promote recovery.

Antihistamines (H₁-receptor antagonists)

CLINICAL PHARMACOLOGY

Common indications	❶ As a first-line treatment for **allergies,** particularly **hay fever** (seasonal allergic rhinitis). ❷ To aid relief of itchiness (**pruritus**) and hives (**urticaria**) due, for example, to insect bites, infections (e.g. chickenpox) and drug allergies. ❸ As an adjunctive treatment in **anaphylaxis,** after administration of <u>adrenaline</u> and other life-saving measures. ❹ Other drugs in this class may be used for **nausea and vomiting** (see <u>Antiemetics, histamine H₁-receptor antagonists</u>).
Mechanisms of action	The term 'antihistamine' is generally used to mean an antagonist of the H₁ receptor. <u>H₂-receptor antagonists</u> have different uses and are discussed separately. Histamine is released from storage granules in mast cells as a result of antigen binding to IgE on the cell surface. Mainly via H₁ receptors, histamine induces the features of immediate-type (type 1) hypersensitivity: increased capillary permeability causing oedema formation (wheal), vasodilatation causing erythema (flare), and itch due to sensory nerve stimulation. When histamine is released in the nasopharynx, as in hay fever, it causes nasal irritation, sneezing, rhinorrhoea, congestion, conjunctivitis and itch. In the skin, it causes urticaria. Widespread histamine release, as in anaphylaxis, produces generalised vasodilatation and vascular leakage, with consequent hypotension. Antihistamines work in these conditions by antagonism at the H₁ receptor, blocking the effects of excess histamine. In anaphylaxis, their effect is too slow to be life-saving, so <u>adrenaline</u> is the more important first-line treatment.
Important adverse effects	The 'first-generation' antihistamines (e.g. chlorphenamine) cause **sedation.** This because histamine, via H₁ receptors, has a role in the brain in maintaining wakefulness. Newer 'second-generation' antihistamines (including loratadine, cetirizine and fexofenadine) do not cross the blood–brain barrier so tend not to have this effect. They have few adverse effects.
Warnings	Commonly used antihistamines, including those mentioned above, are safe in most patients. Sedating antihistamines (e.g. chlorphenamine) should be avoided in ▲**severe liver disease,** as they may precipitate hepatic encephalopathy.
Important interactions	The antihistamines mentioned here are not subject to any major drug interactions.

cetirizine, loratadine, fexofenadine, chlorphenamine

PRACTICAL PRESCRIBING

Prescription	Cetirizine (10 mg tablets), loratadine (10 mg tablets) and chlorphenamine (4 mg tablets and 2 mg/5 mL oral solution) may be purchased without prescription. Cetirizine and loratadine are taken orally on a once daily basis. Chlorphenamine is taken orally every 4–6 hours. In **anaphylaxis,** chlorphenamine 10 mg IV or IM may be administered, but this must not be prioritised over <u>adrenaline</u> and other life-saving measures (e.g. fluid resuscitation).
Administration	There are no special considerations for the administration for cetirizine and loratadine. Although oral chlorphenamine may be taken throughout the day, some patients prefer to reserve it for use in the evening when its sedating effect may be desirable.
Communication	As appropriate, explain that you are offering a treatment to help relieve their allergic symptoms or their itchy rash/hives. In hay fever, the tablets should improve sneezing, itchiness and runniness, but tend not to help with nasal congestion. In the cases of cetirizine and loratadine, you can say that you do not anticipate any side effects. For chlorphenamine, you should mention that it may make them feel sleepy or lose concentration. They should therefore avoid taking it if they need to drive or carry out any other activity that requires concentration. They should also avoid combining it with alcohol, which may exacerbate the effect.
Monitoring	Clinical assessment of allergic symptoms, physical signs (e.g. rash) and enquiry about side effects is the best form of monitoring.
Cost	Non-proprietary antihistamines listed here are inexpensive. Patients who pay for their prescriptions will generally save money if they buy them directly from a pharmacy. There is no reason to use the more expensive brand name products.

Clinical tip—It may be useful to advise patients that larger pack sizes can be obtained if they buy them from the pharmacy counter, rather than off the shelf or from a non-pharmacy retailer. These may be more convenient and economical.

Antimotility drugs

CLINICAL PHARMACOLOGY

Common indications	❶ As a symptomatic treatment for **diarrhoea,** usually in the context of irritable bowel syndrome or viral gastroenteritis.
Mechanisms of action	Loperamide is an opioid that is pharmacologically similar to pethidine. However, unlike pethidine, is does not penetrate the central nervous system (CNS), so has no analgesic effects. It is an **agonist of the opioid μ-receptors in the gastrointestinal tract.** This increases non-propulsive contractions of the gut smooth muscle but reduces propulsive (peristaltic) contractions. As a result, **transit of bowel contents is slowed and anal sphincter tone is increased.** Slower gut transit also allows more time for water absorption, which (in the context of watery diarrhoea) has a desirable effect in hardening the stool. Other opioids (e.g. codeine phosphate) have similar effects but, unless analgesia is also required, there is little reason to prefer them over loperamide.
Important adverse effects	In itself, loperamide is a safe drug with few adverse effects. These are mostly **gastrointestinal effects** predictable from its mechanism of action (e.g. constipation, abdominal cramping and flatulence). Indirectly, adverse effects may arise from the inappropriate inhibition of peristalsis (see Warnings). Where CNS-penetrating opioids are used (e.g. codeine phosphate), there is a risk of opioid toxicity and dependence (see Opioids, weak).
Warnings	Loperamide should be avoided in ▲acute ulcerative colitis where inhibition of peristalsis may increase the risk of megacolon and perforation. For the same reason, it should be avoided where there is a possibility of ▲*Clostridium difficile* colitis, including in patients who develop diarrhoea in association with broad-spectrum antibiotic use (see Clinical tip). It should not be used in ▲acute bloody diarrhoea (dysentery) because this may signify bacterial infection. Particularly worrying in this context is *Escherichia coli*, as certain strains of this can cause a serious condition called haemolytic–uraemic syndrome (HUS). Use of antimotility drugs appears to increase the risk of HUS.
Important interactions	There are no clinically significant interactions.

PRACTICAL PRESCRIBING

Prescription	Loperamide may be purchased over the counter without prescription. In acute 'simple' diarrhoea, the usual dose is 4 mg, followed by 2 mg with each loose stool, generally to a maximum of 8 mg (4 tablets) per day.
Administration	Loperamide is usually taken as a capsule or tablet. A syrup form is available, which may be useful in children (over 4 years old) with acute viral gastroenteritis.
Communication	You should ensure your patient is aware that the only purpose of loperamide is to help settle the diarrhoea. It does nothing for the underlying cause. Make sure they know to stop taking it if they develop constipation, abdominal pain, or (in acute diarrhoea) they find they need to take it for more than 5 days.
Monitoring	The best means of monitoring is to enquire about stool frequency and abdominal symptoms.
Cost	Loperamide is available in non-proprietary form and is inexpensive. Patients who have to pay for their prescriptions will probably save money if they buy it over the counter rather than on prescription.

Clinical tip—Because of the risks of inhibiting peristalsis in the context of *C. difficile* colitis, it is generally unwise to prescribe an antimotility drug for a patient who develops diarrhoea while in hospital. You should at least wait until you have a better idea of its aetiology, such as a positive viral PCR and/or negative *C. difficile* toxin test. Make sure you explain this to the patient, who may be frustrated that while in hospital they cannot get a medicine that, if they were at home, they would simply buy from the chemist.

Antimuscarinics, bronchodilators

CLINICAL PHARMACOLOGY

Common indications	❶ In **chronic obstructive pulmonary disease (COPD),** *short-acting antimuscarinics* are used to relieve breathlessness, e.g. brought on by exercise or during exacerbations. *Long-acting antimuscarinics* (LAMAs) are used to prevent breathlessness and exacerbations. ❷ In **asthma,** *short-acting antimuscarinics* are used as adjuvant treatment for relief of breathlessness during acute exacerbations (added to a short-acting β_2 agonist, e.g. salbutamol). *Long-acting antimuscarinics* are added to high-dose inhaled corticosteroids and long-acting β_2 agonists at 'step 4' in the treatment of chronic asthma.
Mechanisms of action	Antimuscarinic drugs bind to the muscarinic receptor, where they act as a **competitive inhibitor of acetylcholine.** *Stimulation* of the muscarinic receptor brings about a wide range of parasympathetic 'rest and digest' effects. In *blocking* the receptor, antimuscarinics have the opposite effects: they increase heart rate and conduction; **reduce smooth muscle tone,** including in the respiratory tract; and **reduce secretions** from glands in the respiratory and gastrointestinal tracts. In the eye they cause relaxation of the pupillary constrictor and ciliary muscles, causing pupillary dilatation and preventing accommodation, respectively.
Important adverse effects	When antimuscarinic bronchodilators are taken by inhalation, there is relatively little systemic absorption. Adverse effects, apart from **dry mouth,** are uncommon.
Warnings	Antimuscarinics should be used with caution in patients susceptible to ▲**angle-closure glaucoma,** in whom they can precipitate a dangerous rise in intraocular pressure. They should be used with caution in patients with or at risk of arrhythmias. However, in practice, most patients can take these drugs by inhalation without major problems.
Important interactions	Interactions are not generally a problem due to low systemic absorption.

ipratropium, tiotropium, glycopyrronium

PRACTICAL PRESCRIBING

Prescription	*Short-acting antimuscarinics* such as ipratropium are prescribed to be taken four times daily or as needed when the patient feels breathless. They are prescribed at a standard dose (40 micrograms) by inhalation for stable patients, but at a much higher dose (250–500 micrograms 6-hrly) by nebulisation during an acute attack. *Long-acting antimuscarinics* (e.g. tiotropium, glycopyrronium) are prescribed for regular administration, generally once daily.
Administration	Inhaled medication comes in a range of inhaler devices, with the choice of medicine often being directed by the device that best suits the patient. Medication for nebulisation comes as a liquid, which is put into the chamber below a mask covering the mouth and nose of the patient. Oxygen is bubbled through the liquid, vaporising the medicine for the patient to inhale. In patients at risk of carbon dioxide retention, medical air is used in place of oxygen.
Communication	Explain that you are offering a treatment to make their airways relax, which should therefore improve their breathing. They should understand that this treats the symptoms, not the disease. Ensure they are clear on how and when to take the inhaler (e.g. for acute symptoms, pre-emptively before exercise or regularly for long-acting medication). Discuss possible side effects, such as dry mouth, and advise them to chew gum or suck sweets (which should be sugar-free; see <u>Antimuscarinics, genitourinary uses</u>), or keep a bottle of water with them to relieve these.
Monitoring	You should check if the treatment has worked by asking the patient about symptoms and reviewing peak flow measurements (asthma). You should enquire about side effects, particularly dry mouth. You should **check their inhaler technique** every time they are reviewed and correct it as necessary to optimise potential treatment benefits.
Cost	Ipratropium is available in non-proprietary form and is inexpensive. Long-acting antimuscarinics are newer medicines, with most drugs and inhaler devices remaining under patent protection. They are therefore relatively expensive.

Clinical tip—There is no advantage in prescribing short-acting antimuscarinics more than four times daily as this increases adverse effects without increasing benefits. By contrast, β_2 <u>agonists</u> can be administered much more frequently (e.g. 2-hrly) if needed.

Antimuscarinics, cardiovascular and gastrointestinal uses

CLINICAL PHARMACOLOGY

Common indications	❶ Atropine is used first-line in the management of severe or symptomatic **bradycardia** to increase heart rate. ❷ Antimuscarinics (particularly hyoscine butylbromide) are a first-line pharmacological treatment option for **irritable bowel syndrome (IBS)**, where they are used for their antispasmodic effect. ❸ In the care of the dying patient, antimuscarincs (e.g. hyoscine butylbromide) may have a role in reducing **copious respiratory secretions.**
Mechanisms of action	Antimuscarinic drugs bind to the muscarinic receptor, where they act as a **competitive inhibitor of acetylcholine.** *Stimulation* of the muscarinic receptor brings about a wide range of parasympathetic 'rest and digest' effects. In *blocking* the receptor, antimuscarinics have the opposite effects: they **increase heart rate and conduction; reduce smooth muscle tone and peristaltic contraction,** including in the gut and urinary tract; and **reduce secretions** from glands in the respiratory tract and gut. In the eye they cause relaxation of the pupillary constrictor and ciliary muscles, causing pupillary dilatation and preventing accommodation, respectively.
Important adverse effects	Predictably from their antagonism of parasympathetic 'rest and digest' effects, antimuscarinics can cause **tachycardia, dry mouth** and **constipation.** By reducing detrusor muscle activity, they can cause **urinary retention** in patients with benign prostatic hypertrophy. The ocular effects may cause **blurred vision,** especially for near objects. Some antimuscarinics (including atropine) have central effects, which may precipitate **drowsiness** and **confusion,** particularly in the elderly.
Warnings	Antimuscarinics should be used with caution in patients susceptible to ▲**angle-closure glaucoma,** in whom they can precipitate a dangerous rise in intraocular pressure. They should generally be avoided in patients at risk of ▲**arrhythmias** (e.g. those with significant cardiac disease), unless the indication for use is bradycardia.
Important interactions	Adverse effects are more pronounced when they are combined with other drugs that have antimuscarinic effects, such as <u>tricyclic antidepressants</u>.

atropine, hyoscine butylbromide, glycopyrronium

PRACTICAL PRESCRIBING

Prescription	For **bradycardia,** atropine is usually preferred and is given IV in incremental doses (e.g. 300–600 micrograms every 1–2 mins) until an acceptable heart rate is restored. Glycopyrronium is an alternative. It does not penetrate the brain so causes less drowsiness, but it tends not to be readily available on general wards. For **IBS,** an antimuscarinic is taken orally on a regular basis: hyoscine butylbromide (Buscopan®) 10 mg 8-hrly is a common choice. This is available without prescription. For **the control of respiratory secretions,** hyoscine butylbromide or hyoscine hydrobromide is usually given SC, either by injection or as part of a continuous subcutaneous infusion. Note that hyoscine butylbromide or hyoscine hydrobromide have quite different doses – take care that both you and the nursing staff are clear on which one you are using, and that the dose is correct.
Administration	In general, IV administration of atropine should be performed only by, or under direct supervision of, an individual experienced in its use. To facilitate rapid administration in emergencies, atropine is provided in pre-filled disposable syringes. It is a good idea to familiarise yourself with these devices before you need to use them for real. The concentration of atropine in pre-filled syringes may be 100, 200 or 300 micrograms/mL – be sure to check this before administration.
Communication	Depending on the clinical context, it may be appropriate to warn patients about common adverse effects of antimuscarinics, such as dry mouth and blurred vision.
Monitoring	When using antimuscarinics to increase heart rate, high-intensity monitoring (including continuous cardiac rhythm monitoring) is required. It is essential that this is continued after restoration of normal heart rate, as the effect of the drug may only be transient. For other indications, enquiry about symptoms is the best form of monitoring. The dose is titrated to achieve the optimal balance between beneficial and adverse effects.
Cost	Antimuscarinics are relatively inexpensive.

Clinical tip—When treating bradycardia, some practitioners recommend that the initial dose of atropine should be no less than 600 micrograms. This is because, paradoxically, low-dose atropine may transiently *slow* the heart rate before the more predictable positive chronotropic effect supervenes.

Antimuscarinics, genitourinary uses

CLINICAL PHARMACOLOGY

Common indications	❶ To reduce urinary frequency, urgency and urge incontinence in **overactive bladder,** as a first-line pharmacological treatment if bladder training is ineffective.
Mechanisms of action	Antimuscarinic drugs bind to muscarinic receptors, where they act as a **competitive inhibitor of acetylcholine.** Contraction of the smooth muscle of the bladder is under parasympathetic control. Blocking muscarinic receptors therefore **promotes bladder relaxation,** increasing bladder capacity. In patients with overactive bladder, this may **reduce urinary frequency, urgency and urge incontinence.** Antimuscarinics useful in treating overactive bladder tend to be **relatively selective for the M_3 receptor,** which is the main muscarinic receptor subtype in the bladder.
Important adverse effects	Predictably from their antimuscarinic action, **dry mouth** is a very common side effect of these drugs. Other classic antimuscarinic side effects such as **tachycardia, constipation** and **blurred vision** are also common. Urinary retention may occur if there is bladder outflow obstruction.
Warnings	Antimuscarinics are contraindicated in the context of ✘**urinary tract infection.** Urinalysis is therefore an important part of assessment before prescribing treatment for overactive bladder. Central nervous system side effects (drowsiness and confusion) can be particularly problematic in the **elderly** and especially patients with ▲**dementia.** Antimuscarinics should be used with caution in patients susceptible to ▲**angle-closure glaucoma,** in whom they can precipitate a dangerous rise in intraocular pressure. They should be used with caution in patients at risk of ▲**arrhythmias** (e.g. those with significant cardiac disease) and, for obvious reasons, those at risk of ▲**urinary retention.**
Important interactions	Adverse effects are more pronounced when combined with other drugs that have antimuscarinic effects, such as tricyclic antidepressants.

oxybutynin, tolterodine, solifenacin

PRACTICAL PRESCRIBING

Prescription	You should prescribe antimuscarinics for **urge incontinence** only after an adequate trial of bladder retraining. Where they are indicated, an immediate-release form of oxybutynin is recommended for first-line therapy. A typical prescription would be for oxybutynin 5 mg orally every 8 or 12 hours. Other forms of oxybutynin (e.g. modified-release tablets, transdermal patches) and other antimuscarinics should be reserved for use when immediate-release oxybutynin is not tolerated.
Administration	Immediate-release oxybutynin should be taken at roughly equal intervals, with or without food. Modified-release forms should be taken at a similar time each day and swallowed whole, not chewed.
Communication	Explain that you are offering a treatment with a medicine that relaxes the bladder. This will hopefully reduce how often they need to pass water, the urgency with which they need to get to the toilet, and the chance of accidents. Explain that dry mouth is a very common side effect, affecting more than one in ten patients (see Clinical tip). When prescribing for elderly patients it may be prudent to mention that the medicine may cause drowsiness and confusion, and to stop taking it if this occurs.
Monitoring	You should arrange to review your patient within a month of starting therapy to review response and side effects.
Cost	Immediate-release oxybutynin is available in non-proprietary form and is relatively inexpensive. Other preparations are more expensive and should be reserved for second-line use.

Clinical tip—Dry mouth is a very common side effect of antimuscarinic therapy. Patients may find that chewing gum or sucking sweets helps to alleviate this. This may be worth mentioning in your communication with patients, but it is important to say that they should use sugar-free products, because dry mouth increases the risk of tooth decay. For the same reason, good dental care is important for all patients who require antimuscarinic treatment on a long-term basis.

Antipsychotics, first-generation (typical)

CLINICAL PHARMACOLOGY

Common indications	❶ Urgent treatment of severe **psychomotor agitation** that is causing dangerous or violent behaviour, or to calm patients to permit assessment. ❷ **Schizophrenia,** particularly when the metabolic side effects of <u>second-generation (atypical) antipsychotics</u> are likely to be problematic. ❸ **Bipolar disorder,** particularly in acute episodes of mania or hypomania. ❹ **Nausea and vomiting,** particularly in the palliative care setting.
Mechanisms of action	Antipsychotic drugs **block post-synaptic dopamine D_2 receptors.** There are three main dopaminergic pathways in the central nervous system. The *mesolimbic/mesocortical pathway* runs between the midbrain and the limbic system/frontal cortex. D_2 blockade in this pathway is probably the main determinant of antipsychotic effect, but this is incompletely understood. The *nigrostriatal pathway* connects the substantia nigra with the corpus striatum of the basal ganglia. The *tuberohypophyseal pathway* connects the hypothalamus with the pituitary gland. D_2 receptors are also found in the *chemoreceptor trigger zone*, where blockade accounts for their use in nausea and vomiting. All antipsychotics, but particularly chlorpromazine, have some sedative effect. This may be beneficial in the context of acute psychomotor agitation.
Important adverse effects	**Extrapyramidal effects** – movement abnormalities that arise from D_2 blockade in the *nigrostriatal pathway* – are the main drawback of first-generation antipsychotics. They take several forms: **acute dystonic reactions** are involuntary parkinsonian movements or muscle spasms; **akathisia** is a state of inner restlessness; and **neuroleptic malignant syndrome** is rare but life-threatening side effect characterised by rigidity, confusion, autonomic dysregulation and pyrexia. These all tend to occur early in treatment. By contrast, **tardive dyskinesia** is a late adverse effect (*tardive*, late), occurring after months or years of therapy. This comprises movements that are pointless, involuntary and repetitive (e.g. lip smacking). It is disabling and may not resolve on stopping treatment. Other adverse effects include **drowsiness, hypotension, QT-interval prolongation** (and consequent **arrhythmias**), **erectile dysfunction,** and symptoms arising from **hyperprolactinaemia** due to *tuberohypophyseal* D_2 blockade (e.g. menstrual disturbance, galactorrhoea and breast pain).
Warnings	▲**Elderly** patients are particularly sensitive to antipsychotics, so start with lower doses. Antipsychotics should ideally be avoided in ▲**dementia,** as they may increase the risk of death and stroke. They should be avoided if possible in ▲**Parkinson's disease** due to their extrapyramidal effects.
Important interactions	Consult the BNF when prescribing for a patient taking antipsychotics as there is an extensive list of interactions. Prominent among these are ▲**drugs that prolong the QT interval** (e.g. <u>amiodarone</u>, <u>macrolides</u>).

PRACTICAL PRESCRIBING

Prescription	Regular treatment is required to treat schizophrenia and should only be started or adjusted under the guidance of a psychiatrist. A single dose may be used to control acute or violent behaviour. A common choice is haloperidol 0.5–3.0 mg IM, although higher doses may be used in extreme cases. This should be given only under guidance of an appropriately experienced clinician. For the control of nausea, haloperidol is used in regular small oral or SC doses (e.g. 1.5 mg at night) or as a component of a continuous SC infusion.
Administration	For regular administration, typical antipsychotics can be taken orally (tablet and liquid) or given by slow-release IM ('depot') injection.
	In emergencies, haloperidol is usually given by rapid-acting IM injection and occasionally IV for rapid control of symptoms, although it is not licensed by this route. Intravenous haloperidol should only be administered by clinicians capable of managing neurological and cardiovascular side effects including arrhythmias such as torsade de pointes (a form of ventricular tachycardia), which are more likely when antipsychotics are given by injection or in high dose.
Communication	Adherence is a significant issue when treating psychiatric disorders, both because of the underlying disease and adverse effects of treatment. Good communication with your patient about the aims and benefits of treatment, as well as its potential side effects, are therefore very important. It is also important to emphasise that patients should report that they are taking antipsychotics to other healthcare professionals involved in their care, as many other medicines can interfere with the way they work.
Monitoring	The aim of treatment with antipsychotics is control of symptoms, so frequent reviews of symptoms and signs are important. The antipsychotic effects may take several weeks to become established and the dose may need to be adjusted to obtain the optimum balance between beneficial and adverse effects. When using high doses for acute control of psychotic/violent behaviour the dose–response relationship is unpredictable, so you should ensure that appropriate monitoring is available to detect neurological, respiratory and cardiovascular depression.
Cost	Typical antipsychotics are relatively old drugs and are available in inexpensive non-proprietary forms. Branded products, including oral solutions and depot injections, are more expensive.

Clinical tip—Haloperidol is also licensed for the treatment of intractable hiccups!

Antipsychotics, second-generation (atypical)

CLINICAL PHARMACOLOGY

Common indications	❶ Urgent treatment of severe **psychomotor agitation** leading to dangerous or violent behaviour, or to calm such patients to permit assessment. ❷ **Schizophrenia,** particularly when extrapyramidal side effects have complicated the use of first-generation (typical) antipsychotics, or when negative symptoms are prominent. ❸ **Bipolar disorder,** particularly in acute episodes of mania or hypomania.
Mechanisms of action	Antipsychotic drugs **block post-synaptic dopamine D₂ receptors.** There are three main dopaminergic pathways in the central nervous system. The *mesolimbic/mesocortical pathway* runs between the midbrain and the limbic system/frontal cortex. D_2 blockade in this pathway is probably the main determinant of antipsychotic effect, but this is incompletely understood. The *nigrostriatal pathway* connects the substantia nigra with the corpus striatum of the basal ganglia. The *tuberohypophyseal pathway* connects the hypothalamus with the pituitary gland. Features that distinguish second-generation antipsychotics from first-generation agents are improved efficacy in 'treatment-resistant' schizophrenia (particularly true of clozapine) and against negative symptoms, and a lower risk of extrapyramidal symptoms. Possible mechanisms for these differences include a higher affinity for **other receptors** (particularly 5-HT$_{2A}$ receptors), and a characteristic of **'looser' binding** to the D_2 receptors (in the case of clozapine and quetiapine).
Important adverse effects	Most antipsychotics cause some degree of **sedation.** Blocking dopamine in the *nigrostriatal pathway* may produce movement abnormalities called **extrapyramidal effects.** These are more common with first-generation antipsychotics, where they are discussed more fully. **Metabolic disturbance,** including weight gain, diabetes mellitus and lipid changes, is a common problem with second-generation antipsychotics. Antipsychotics can **prolong the QT interval** and thus cause **arrhythmias.** Risperidone has particular effects on dopaminergic transmission in the *tuberohypophyseal pathway,* which regulates secretion of prolactin. This can cause **breast symptoms** (in both women and men) and **sexual dysfunction.** Clozapine causes a severe deficiency of neutrophils **(agranulocytosis)** in about 1% of patients, and rarely causes **myocarditis.**
Warnings	Antipsychotics should be used with caution in patients with ▲**cardiovascular disease.** Clozapine must not be used in patients with ✘**severe heart disease** or a history of ✘**neutropenia.**
Important interactions	Sedation may be more pronounced when used with other sedating drugs. They should not be combined with other ▲dopamine-blocking antiemetics and ▲**drugs that prolong the QT interval** (e.g. amiodarone, quinine, macrolides, selective serotonin reuptake inhibitors).

quetiapine, olanzapine, risperidone, clozapine

PRACTICAL PRESCRIBING

Prescription	Decisions to start treatment with a second-generation antipsychotic drug should be taken by a specialist. They may be used both for treatment of acute symptoms and for prevention of subsequent attacks. Options include daily oral treatment or intermittent slow-release IM ('depot') injections. Clozapine is considered when other agents have proved ineffective or intolerable. You are most likely to encounter these drugs in patients already established on treatment, for example when they are admitted to hospital. In this situation you should not usually stop them, but must check carefully that the acute illness is not caused by the antipsychotic, that it does not present a contraindication to antipsychotic treatment, and that any new drugs introduced do not interact with the antipsychotic.
Administration	Oral antipsychotic medications are best taken at bedtime.
Communication	When you encounter patients established on antipsychotic treatment, it is worth reminding them that they should always inform any healthcare professional involved in their care what treatment they are on. This is particularly important for antipsychotics as many other medicines can interfere with the way they work. Patients taking clozapine should know about the need for regular blood test monitoring and of the need to report infective symptoms immediately.
Monitoring	Assessment of symptoms and signs is the best form of monitoring for treatment efficacy. For most antipsychotics, blood tests (typically full blood count, renal and liver profiles) are required at the start of treatment and periodically thereafter; an intensive monitoring programme is required for clozapine due to the risk of agranulocytosis. Monitoring for metabolic and cardiovascular side effects is important for second-generation antipsychotics. This includes measurement of weight, lipid profile and fasting blood glucose at baseline and intermittently during treatment.
Cost	Non-proprietary forms of quetiapine, olanzapine and risperidone are available and are substantially less expensive than their brand name counterparts.

Clinical tip—When you see a patient in hospital who is taking an antipsychotic drug, always check the QT-interval on their ECG. Most antipsychotics can lengthen this to some extent (which presents a risk of dangerous arrhythmias), and this may be exacerbated by drugs administered for the acute problem (e.g. macrolide antibiotics for infection).

Aspirin

CLINICAL PHARMACOLOGY

Common indications	❶ For treatment of **acute coronary syndrome** and **acute ischaemic stroke,** where rapid inhibition of platelet aggregation can prevent or limit arterial thrombosis and reduce subsequent mortality. ❷ For long-term secondary prevention of thrombotic arterial events in patients with **cardiovascular, cerebrovascular** and **peripheral arterial disease.** ❸ To reduce the risk of intracardiac thrombus and embolic stroke in **atrial fibrillation** where warfarin and novel oral anticoagulants are contraindicated. ❹ To control **mild-to-moderate pain and fever** (see Non-steroidal anti-inflammatory drugs, although other drugs are usually preferred, particularly in patients with inflammatory conditions).
Mechanisms of action	Thrombotic events occur when platelet-rich thrombus forms in atheromatous arteries and occludes the circulation. Aspirin **irreversibly inhibits cyclooxygenase** (COX) to reduce production of the pro-aggregatory factor thromboxane from arachidonic acid, **reducing platelet aggregation** and the risk of arterial occlusion. The antiplatelet effect of aspirin occurs at **low doses** and lasts for the lifetime of a platelet (which does not have a nucleus to allow synthesis of new COX) and thus only wears off as new platelets are made.
Important adverse effects	The most common adverse effect of aspirin is **gastrointestinal irritation.** More serious effects include **gastrointestinal ulceration** and **haemorrhage** and hypersensitivity reactions including **bronchospasm.** In regular high-dose therapy aspirin causes **tinnitus.** Aspirin is life-threatening in **overdose.** Features include hyperventilation, hearing changes, metabolic acidosis and confusion, followed by convulsions, cardiovascular collapse and respiratory arrest.
Warnings	Aspirin should not be given to ✖**children aged under 16 years** due to the risk of **Reye's syndrome,** a rare but life-threatening illness that principally affects the liver and brain. It should not be taken by people with ✖**aspirin hypersensitivity,** i.e. who have had bronchospasm or other allergic symptoms triggered by exposure to aspirin or another NSAID. However, aspirin is not *routinely* contraindicated in asthma. Aspirin should be avoided in the ✖**third trimester of pregnancy** when prostaglandin inhibition may lead to premature closure of the ductus arteriosus. Aspirin should be used with caution in people with ▲**peptic ulceration** (e.g. prescribe gastroprotection) or ▲**gout,** as it may trigger an acute attack.
Important interactions	Aspirin acts synergistically with other antiplatelet agents, which although therapeutically beneficial can lead to increased risk of bleeding. Thus, although it may be given with ▲**antiplatelet drugs** (e.g. clopidogrel, dipyridamole) and ▲**anticoagulants** (e.g. heparin, warfarin) in some situations (e.g. acute coronary syndrome), caution is required.

PRACTICAL PRESCRIBING

Prescription	Aspirin is available for oral or rectal (higher doses) administration. In **acute coronary syndrome,** prescribe aspirin initially as a once-only *loading dose* of 300 mg followed by a regular dose of 75 mg daily. For **acute ischaemic stroke,** prescribe aspirin 300 mg daily for 2 weeks before switching to 75 mg daily. For **long-term prevention of thrombosis** after an acute event or in people with atrial fibrillation, prescribe low-dose aspirin 75 mg daily. Much higher doses of aspirin are required for the treatment of **pain,** with a maximum daily dose of 4 g, taken in divided doses. **Gastroprotection** (e.g. omeprazole 20 mg daily, see <u>Proton pump inhibitors</u>) should be considered for patients taking low-dose aspirin who are at increased risk of gastrointestinal complications. Risk factors include age >65 years, previous peptic ulcer disease, comorbidities (such as cardiovascular disease, diabetes), and concurrent therapy with other drugs with gastrointestinal side effects, particularly NSAIDs and <u>prednisolone</u>.
Administration	In order to minimise gastric irritation, aspirin should be taken after food. Enteric-coated tablets may help further, but are associated with slower absorption and therefore not suitable for use in medical emergencies or for rapid pain relief.
Communication	Advise patients that the purpose of low-dose aspirin treatment is to prevent heart attacks or strokes and to prolong life. Warn them to watch out for indigestion or bleeding symptoms and report these to their doctor if they occur.
Monitoring	Enquiry about side effects is the most appropriate form of monitoring.
Cost	Aspirin is inexpensive, available off-patent and over the counter.

Clinical tip—In the UK, aspirin is not recommended or licensed for use in primary prevention (i.e. in patients who have not previously had a vascular event). The reason is that large-scale randomised-controlled trials and meta-analyses have found that the absolute risk of serious vascular events in this group is low (around 1/500), and any potential benefits of low-dose aspirin are offset by the increased risk of serious bleeding (around 1/1000).

Benzodiazepines

CLINICAL PHARMACOLOGY

Common indications

❶ In the first-line management of **seizures** and **status epilepticus.**
❷ In the first-line management of **alcohol withdrawal reactions.**
❸ As a common choice for **sedation for interventional procedures,** if general anaesthesia is unnecessary or undesirable.
❹ For *short-term* treatment of severe, disabling or distressing **anxiety.**
❺ For *short-term* treatment of severe, disabling or distressing **insomnia.**

Mechanisms of action

The target of benzodiazepines is the γ-aminobutyric acid type A (GABA$_A$) receptor. The GABA$_A$ receptor is a chloride channel that opens in response to binding by GABA, the main inhibitory neurotransmitter in the brain. Opening the channel allows chloride to flow into the cell, making the cell more resistant to depolarisation. **Benzodiazepines facilitate and enhance binding of GABA to the GABA$_A$ receptor.** This has a widespread depressant effect on synaptic transmission. The clinical manifestations of this include reduced anxiety, sleepiness, sedation and anticonvulsive effects. Ethanol ('alcohol') also acts on the GABA$_A$ receptor, and in chronic excessive use the patient becomes tolerant to its presence. Abrupt cessation then provokes the excitatory state of **alcohol withdrawal.** This can be treated by introducing a benzodiazepine, which can then be withdrawn in a gradual and more controlled way.

Important adverse effects

Predictably, benzodiazepines cause dose-dependent **drowsiness, sedation** and **coma.** There is relatively little cardiorespiratory depression in **benzodiazepine overdose** (in contrast to opioid overdose), but loss of airway reflexes can lead to **airway obstruction** and **death.** If used repeatedly for more than a few weeks, a state of **dependence** can develop. Abrupt cessation then produces a **withdrawal reaction** similar to that seen with alcohol.

Warnings

The ▲**elderly** are more susceptible to the effects of benzodiazepines so should receive a lower dose. Benzodiazepines are best avoided in patients with significant ▲**respiratory impairment** or ▲**neuromuscular disease** (e.g. myasthenia gravis). They should also be avoided in ▲**liver failure** as they may precipitate hepatic encephalopathy; if their use is essential (e.g. for alcohol withdrawal), lorazepam may be the best choice, as it depends less on the liver for its elimination.

Important interactions

The effects of benzodiazepines are additive to those of other sedating drugs, including alcohol and opioids. Most depend on cytochrome P450 enzymes for elimination, so concurrent use with ▲**cytochrome P450 inhibitors** (e.g. amiodarone, diltiazem, macrolides, fluconazole, protease inhibitors) may increase their effects.

diazepam, temazepam, lorazepam, chlordiazepoxide, midazolam

PRACTICAL PRESCRIBING

Prescription	The effects of the various benzodiazepines are similar. What distinguishes them is their *duration of action*, and this dictates how they are used. For **seizures,** a long-acting drug is preferred, usually lorazepam (initial dose 4 mg IV) or diazepam (10 mg IV). Diazepam can also be given rectally for seizures, but you must use the rectal solution (rather than suppositories) to ensure rapid absorption. For **alcohol withdrawal,** oral chlordiazepoxide (also long-acting) is the traditional choice, but diazepam is probably equally acceptable; the dosage regimen depends on the patient's symptoms and their usual alcohol intake. In **sedation for interventional procedures,** a short-acting drug is best, as this allows rapid recovery after completion of the procedure or inadvertent over-sedation. Midazolam is most appropriate here, but it should only be used by individuals skilled in safe sedation practice. For **insomnia** and **anxiety,** an intermediate-acting drug (e.g. temazepam 10 mg orally at bedtime) is generally preferred.
Administration	Diazepam is available as a water-based solution and an oil-in-water emulsion. The solution is more irritant to veins. Intravenous administration of benzodiazepines, whether for seizures or sedation, should be undertaken only where facilities and expertise exist to deal with over-sedation (including capabilities for airway management). They should be injected slowly.
Communication	When treating **insomnia** and **anxiety,** advise your patient that pharmacological therapy is only a short-term measure. Discuss the risks of dependence, advising that this can be minimised by avoiding daily use if possible and taking them for no longer than 4 weeks. Advise patients that they should not drive or operate complex or heavy machinery after taking the drug, and caution them that sometimes sleepiness may persist the following day.
Monitoring	Close monitoring of the patient's clinical status and vital signs are essential following IV or high-dose oral administration of a benzodiazepine, including the settings of **seizures, alcohol withdrawal** and **sedation.** In **insomnia** and **anxiety,** enquiry about symptoms and side effects is the best form of monitoring.
Cost	Benzodiazepines are generally inexpensive.

Clinical tip—Flumazenil is a specific antagonist of benzodiazepines. However, use of this drug is rarely indicated. Specifically, it should *not* be given to reverse benzodiazepine-induced sedation when this forms part of a mixed or uncertain overdose. In this context, flumazenil may precipitate seizures which – having now blocked the benzodiazepine receptor – will be difficult to treat.

Beta$_2$-agonists

CLINICAL PHARMACOLOGY

Common indications	**❶ Asthma:** short-acting β$_2$-agonists are used to relieve breathlessness. Long-acting β$_2$-agonists are used as 'step 3' treatment for chronic asthma, but must *always* be given in combination with <u>inhaled corticosteroids</u>. **❷ Chronic obstructive pulmonary disease (COPD):** short-acting β$_2$-agonists are used to relieve breathlessness. Long-acting β$_2$-agonists are an option for second-line therapy of COPD. **❸ Hyperkalaemia:** nebulised salbutamol may be used as an additional treatment (alongside <u>insulin</u>, <u>glucose</u> and <u>calcium gluconate</u>) for the urgent treatment of a high serum potassium concentration.
Mechanisms of action	Beta$_2$-receptors are found in smooth muscle of the bronchi, gastrointestinal tract, uterus and blood vessels. Stimulation of this G protein-coupled receptor activates a signalling cascade that leads to **smooth muscle relaxation.** This improves airflow in constricted airways, reducing the symptoms of breathlessness. Like insulin, β$_2$-agonists also **stimulate Na$^+$/K$^+$-ATPase pumps** on cell surface membranes, thereby **causing a shift of K$^+$ from the extracellular to intracellular compartment.** This makes them a useful adjunct in the treatment of **hyperkalaemia,** particularly when IV access is difficult. However, their effect is less reliable than other therapies, so they should not be used in isolation. Beta$_2$-agonists are classified as short-acting (salbutamol, terbutaline) or long-acting (salmeterol, formoterol) according to their duration of effect.
Important adverse effects	Activation of β$_2$-receptors in other tissues accounts for the common 'fight or flight' adverse effects of **tachycardia, palpitations, anxiety** and **tremor.** They also promote glycogenolysis, so may increase the serum glucose concentration. At high doses, serum lactate levels may also rise. Long-acting β$_2$-agonists can cause **muscle cramps**.
Warnings	Long-acting β$_2$-agonists should be used in asthma only if an <u>inhaled corticosteroid</u> is also part of therapy. This is because, without a steroid, long-acting β$_2$-agonists are associated with increased asthma deaths. Care should be taken when prescribing β$_2$-agonists for patients with ▲**cardiovascular disease,** in whom tachycardia may provoke angina or arrhythmias. This is especially pertinent in the treatment of hyperkalaemia, when high doses may be necessary.
Important interactions	<u>Beta-blockers</u> may reduce the effectiveness of β$_2$-agonists. Concomitant use of high-dose nebulised β$_2$-agonists with theophylline and <u>corticosteroids</u> can lead to hypokalaemia, so serum potassium concentrations should be monitored.

salbutamol, salmeterol, formoterol, terbutaline

PRACTICAL PRESCRIBING

Prescription	Inhaled short-acting β_2-agonists are prescribed for 'as required' administration. A common choice in adults is salbutamol 100–200 micrograms inhaled as required. In asthma and COPD exacerbations requiring hospital treatment, nebulised therapy is more often used (e.g. salbutamol 2.5 mg nebulised 4-hrly; see Clinical tip), although inhalation via a spacer is reasonable provided the exacerbation is not life threatening. Long-acting β_2-agonists are used for maintenance therapy and are therefore prescribed regularly (usually twice daily). To assure co-administration with a steroid in asthma, they may be prescribed as part of a combination inhaler (e.g. Symbicort® or Seretide®, usually prescribed by brand name). These combinations are also used in COPD, where they can improve convenience.
Administration	Inhaled medication is administered by a range of devices, with choice of medicine often being directed by the device that best suits the patient. Drugs are delivered in **aerosol** (metered dose inhaler [MDI]) or **dry powder** form. Provision of a **spacer with metered dose inhalers** can improve airway deposition and treatment efficacy and reduce oral adverse effects. The patient should be trained how to use their **inhaler** and **technique** should be checked and corrected at every consultation.
Communication	Explain that the medicine will make their airways relax and therefore improve their breathing. Make sure that they understand that this treats the symptoms, not the disease. Consequently, if they find themselves needing to use the β_2-agonists very frequently, then they should seek medical advice, or increase their other treatment (e.g. inhaled corticosteroid) in accordance with a written action plan. Make sure that they are clear on how and when to take the inhaler (e.g. for acute symptoms, pre-emptively before exercise or regularly for long-acting medication).
Monitoring	Patients with asthma can monitor their disease severity through their symptoms and by serial measurements of peak expiratory flow rate. They may be able to adjust their own treatment with guidance from their action plan. Likewise, symptom severity and exacerbation rates are the main indicators of effect in COPD.
Cost	Non-proprietary versions of short-acting β_2-agonists are relatively inexpensive. However, long-acting β_2-agonists, particularly as part of combination inhalers, are costly. Together, Seretide® and Symbicort® prescriptions cost NHS England more than £500m per annum.

Clinical tip—When prescribing nebuliser therapy, you should always indicate whether the nebuliser should be driven by oxygen or air. In general, oxygen should be used in asthma, whereas medical air should be used in COPD, due to the risk of CO_2 retention.

Beta-blockers

CLINICAL PHARMACOLOGY

Common indications	❶ **Ischaemic heart disease:** as a first-line option to improve symptoms and prognosis associated with **angina** and **acute coronary syndrome.** ❷ **Chronic heart failure:** as a first-line option to improve prognosis. ❸ **Atrial fibrillation:** as a first-line option to reduce the ventricular rate and, in paroxysmal atrial fibrillation, to maintain sinus rhythm. ❹ **Supraventricular tachycardia (SVT):** as a first-line option in patients without circulatory compromise to restore sinus rhythm. ❺ **Hypertension:** although not generally indicated for initial therapy, they may be used when other medicines (e.g. calcium channel blockers, ACE inhibitors, thiazide diuretics) are insufficient or inappropriate.
Mechanisms of action	Beta₁-adrenoreceptors are located mainly in the heart, whereas β₂-adrenoreceptors are found mostly in smooth muscle of blood vessels and the airways. Via the β₁-receptor, **β-blockers reduce force of contraction and speed of conduction in the heart.** This relieves myocardial ischaemia by reducing cardiac work and oxygen demand, and increasing myocardial perfusion. They improve prognosis in heart failure by 'protecting' the heart from the effects of chronic sympathetic stimulation. They slow the ventricular rate in atrial fibrillation mainly by **prolonging the refractory period of the atrioventricular (AV) node.** SVT often involves a self-perpetuating ('re-entry') circuit that takes in the AV node; β-blockers may break this and restore sinus rhythm. In hypertension, β-blockers lower blood pressure through a variety of means, one of which is by **reducing renin secretion** from the kidney, since this is mediated by β₁-receptors.
Important adverse effects	Beta-blockers commonly cause fatigue, cold extremities, headache and gastrointestinal disturbance (e.g. nausea). They can cause sleep disturbance and nightmares. They may cause impotence in men.
Warnings	In patients with ✖**asthma,** β-blockers can cause life-threatening bronchospasm and should be avoided. This effect is mediated by blockade of β₂-adrenoreceptors in the airways. Beta-blockers are usually safe in **chronic obstructive pulmonary disease,** although it is prudent to choose a β-blocker that is relatively β₁-selective (e.g. atenolol, bisoprolol, metoprolol), rather than non-selective (e.g. propranolol). When used in ▲**heart failure,** β-blockers should be started at a low dose and increased slowly, as they may initially impair cardiac function. They should be avoided in patients with ▲**haemodynamic instability** and are contraindicated in ✖**heart block.** Beta-blockers generally require dosage reduction in significant ▲**hepatic failure.**
Important interactions	Beta-blockers must not be used with ✖non-dihydropyridine calcium channel blockers (e.g. verapamil, diltiazem). This combination can cause heart failure, bradycardia, and even asystole.

bisoprolol, atenolol, propranolol, metoprolol

PRACTICAL PRESCRIBING

Prescription	Beta-blockers are usually prescribed orally as part of the patient's regular medication. Dosage varies according to the drug and the indication – the starting dose in heart failure is lower than that for ischaemic heart disease or hypertension. It is generally best to start at the lowest dosage listed in the BNF for that indication. Intravenous preparations (e.g. of metoprolol) are available for use when rapid effect is necessary.
Administration	Orally administered β-blockers should be taken at equal intervals (e.g. roughly the same time each day for once daily drugs such as bisoprolol); the exact time is not important. Intravenous preparations should be prescribed and administered only by those experienced in their use, and only in a closely monitored environment.
Communication	Explain the rationale for treatment as appropriate for the situation. Discuss common side effects, including impotence where relevant. Warn patients with heart failure about the risk of initial deterioration in their symptoms, and advise them to seek medical attention if this occurs. Warn patients with obstructive airways disease to stop treatment and seek medical advice if they develop any breathing difficulty.
Monitoring	The best guide to dosage adjustment is the patient's symptoms (e.g. chest pain) and heart rate (in ischaemic heart disease, aim for a resting heart rate of around 55–60 beats/min).
Cost	Atenolol, bisoprolol and metoprolol are all available in non-proprietary forms, and are relatively inexpensive. Modified-release metoprolol is only available as a branded product and is significantly more expensive, so should be used only where there is a compelling reason to do so.

Clinical tip—When starting a β-blocker acutely, such as in acute coronary syndrome, it is usually best to select a drug with a relatively short half-life, e.g. standard-release oral metoprolol (typical starting dose 12.5 mg 8-hrly; later increased to 25 mg 8-hrly). This will be more responsive to dosage adjustment and can be stopped quickly if necessary. It can be converted to a once daily preparation (e.g. bisoprolol 10 mg daily) for long-term use.

Bisphosphonates

CLINICAL PHARMACOLOGY

Common indications	❶ Alendronic acid is used as the first-line drug treatment option for patients at risk of **osteoporotic fragility fractures.** ❷ Pamidronate and zoledronic acid are used in the treatment of **severe hypercalcaemia of malignancy** after appropriate intravenous rehydration. ❸ For patients with **myeloma** and **breast cancer with bone metastases,** pamidronate and zoledronic acid reduce the risk of pathological fractures, cord compression and the need for radiotherapy or surgery. ❹ Bisphosphonates are used first-line in the treatment of metabolically-active **Paget's disease,** with the aim of reducing bone turnover and pain.
Mechanisms of action	Bisphosphonates reduce bone turnover by inhibiting the action of osteoclasts, the cells responsible for bone resorption. Bisphosphonates have a similar structure to naturally occurring pyrophosphate, hence are readily incorporated into bone. As bone is resorbed, bisphosphonates accumulate in osteoclasts, where they inhibit activity and promote apoptosis. The net effect is reduction in bone loss and improvement in bone mass.
Important adverse effects	Common side effects include **oesophagitis** (when taken orally) and **hypophosphataemia.** A rare but serious adverse effect of bisphosphonates is **osteonecrosis of the jaw,** which is more likely with high-dose IV therapy. Good dental care is important to minimise the risk of this. Another rare but important adverse effect is **atypical femoral fracture,** particularly in patients on long-term treatment.
Warnings	Bisphosphonates are renally excreted and should be avoided in ✖**severe renal impairment.** They are contraindicated in the context of ✖**hypocalcaemia.** Oral administration is contraindicated in patients with active ✖**upper gastrointestinal disorders.** Because of the risk of jaw osteonecrosis, care should be exercised in prescribing bisphosphonates for ▲**smokers** and patients with major ▲**dental disease.**
Important interactions	Bisphosphonates bind calcium. Their absorption is therefore reduced if taken with <u>calcium</u> salts (including milk), as well as <u>antacids</u> and <u>iron</u> salts (see Administration).

alendronic acid, disodium pamidronate, zoledronic acid

PRACTICAL PRESCRIBING

Prescription	For **osteoporosis,** alendronic acid is prescribed orally, 70 mg once weekly. For severe **hypercalcaemia** and **bone metastases,** pamidronate or zoledronic acid are prescribed as slow IV infusions, in single or divided doses. Calcium-lowering effects may not become apparent for 3–4 days and are maximal at 7–10 days, so re-prescription should not be considered before 1 week. For **Paget's disease,** risedronate is given orally and pamidronate as an IV infusion.
Administration	Oral bisphosphonates are poorly absorbed, but this can be enhanced by correct administration. For example, alendronic acid tablets should be swallowed whole at least 30 minutes before breakfast or other medications, taken with plenty of water. The patient should remain upright for 30 minutes after taking to reduce oesophageal irritation.
Communication	Explain that you are recommending a medicine to help strengthen the bones to prevent fractures and/or lower calcium levels in the blood to improve symptoms. Explain that the tablets can cause inflammation of the gullet. To minimise this risk, give clear advice on how to take the tablets and ask them to report any symptoms of oesophageal irritation. Advise patients to see their dentist before and during bisphosphonate treatment. Emphasise the dose and frequency of bisphosphonate treatment to avoid overdosing errors.
Monitoring	In **osteoporosis,** check and replace calcium and vitamin D before treatment. Monitor efficacy using dual-energy X-ray absorptiometry (DEXA) scans every 1–2 years to check bone density is stable or increasing. For **hypercalcaemia,** monitor efficacy by symptom enquiry and reduction in calcium levels. In the treatment of **myeloma, bone metastases** and **Paget's disease,** enquire about symptoms (e.g. bone pain) and bone complications (e.g. pathological fracture). For **safety,** be alert to symptoms of oesophagitis, osteonecrosis of the jaw and atypical femoral fractures, and monitor calcium and phosphate.
Cost	Alendronic acid is the cheapest bisphosphonate; non-proprietary preparations cost around £1 a month. Pamidronate costs around £100 a month for Paget's disease and zoledronic acid (currently branded preparations only) costs around £175 a month for bone metastases.

Clinical tip—Fragility fractures cause significant morbidity and mortality. After hip fracture, 30% die within 1 year and 50% are left with loss of function. Bisphosphonates reduce recurrent fracture by 50%. You can assume a diagnosis of osteoporosis in women aged >75 years who have had a fragility fracture, and start treatment with a bisphosphonate without need for further investigation for osteoporosis, i.e. do not do a DEXA scan.

Calcium and vitamin D

CLINICAL PHARMACOLOGY

Common indications	❶ Calcium and vitamin D are used in **osteoporosis** to ensure positive calcium balance when dietary intake and/or sunlight exposure is insufficient. Other treatments, such as <u>bisphosphonates</u>, may be given to reduce the risk of fragility fractures. ❷ Calcium and vitamin D are used in **chronic kidney disease** to treat and prevent secondary hyperparathyroidism and renal osteodystrophy. ❸ Calcium (as *calcium gluconate*) is used in **severe hyperkalaemia** to prevent life-threatening arrhythmias. Other treatments, e.g. <u>insulin</u> with <u>glucose</u>, are given to lower the potassium concentration. ❹ Calcium is used in **hypocalcaemia** that is symptomatic (e.g. paraesthesia, tetany, seizures) or severe (<1.9 mmol/L). ❺ Vitamin D is used in the prevention and treatment of **vitamin D deficiency,** including for rickets (in children) and osteomalacia (adults).
Mechanisms of action	Calcium is essential for normal function of muscle, nerves, bone and clotting. Calcium homeostasis is controlled by parathyroid hormone and vitamin D, which increase serum calcium levels and bone mineralisation, and calcitonin which reduces serum calcium levels. In **osteoporosis** there is a loss of bone mass which increases the risk of fracture. Restoring positive calcium balance either by dietary means or by administering calcium and vitamin D may reduce the rate of bone loss; whether this prevents fractures is less clear. In severe **chronic kidney disease,** impaired phosphate excretion and reduced activation of vitamin D cause hyperphosphataemia and hypocalcaemia. This stimulates secondary hyperparathyroidism, which leads to a range of bone changes called renal osteodystrophy. Treatment may include oral calcium supplements to bind phosphate in the gut, and alfacalcidol to provide vitamin D that does not depend on renal activation. In **hyperkalaemia,** calcium raises the myocardial threshold potential, reducing excitability and the risk of arrhythmias. It has no effect on the serum potassium level. The rationale for the use of calcium in **hypocalcaemia** and vitamin D in **vitamin D deficiency** is self-explanatory.
Important adverse effects	Oral calcium is usually well tolerated, but may cause **dyspepsia** and **constipation.** When administered IV for the treatment of hyperkalaemia, calcium gluconate can cause **cardiovascular collapse** if administered too fast, and **local tissue damage** if accidentally given into subcutaneous tissue.
Warnings	Calcium and vitamin D should be avoided in ✖**hypercalcaemia.**
Important interactions	Oral calcium reduces the absorption of many drugs including <u>iron</u>, <u>bisphosphonates</u>, <u>tetracyclines</u> and <u>levothyroxine</u>. Administered IV, calcium must not be allowed to mix with ✖sodium bicarbonate due to the risk of precipitation.

calcium carbonate, calcium gluconate, colecalciferol, alfacalcidol

PRACTICAL PRESCRIBING

Prescription	In **osteoporosis,** you should aim to supplement dietary intake with 1–1.2 g of calcium and 800 units of vitamin D per day. Various combined preparations of calcium and vitamin D are available; a common choice is Adcal D$_3$® two tablets daily (each tablet contains calcium 600 mg and colecalciferol 400 units). In **severe hyperkalaemia,** you should prescribe 10 mL of calcium gluconate 10% for administration by slow IV injection. Repeat doses may be required if ECG changes persist. Given the urgency of the situation, it is acceptable to administer the treatment first and write the prescription later. You should **seek expert guidance** for the management of severe or symptomatic hypocalcaemia; vitamin D deficiency; and in the use of calcium and vitamin D in severe chronic kidney disease.
Administration	**Oral calcium** preparations should usually be chewed then swallowed. Doses should be separated from potentially interacting medicines (see Important interactions) by about 4 hours. They may also interact with certain foods, including spinach, bananas and whole cereals; about 2 hours' separation is required if these have been consumed. **Calcium gluconate** should be administered by slow IV injection over 5–10 minutes into a large vein. Make sure the cannula is working by first flushing it with sodium chloride 0.9%, in order to avoid accidental subcutaneous administration ('extravasation').
Communication	Explain the rationale for treatment as appropriate for the clinical indication. Advise patients to seek medical advice if they develop side effects such as abdominal pain and limb pain, as these may be a sign of high calcium levels, requiring a blood test.
Monitoring	Patients with severe hyperkalaemia require continuous cardiac monitoring. You should repeat a 12-lead ECG after administration of calcium gluconate to confirm resolution of initial ECG abnormalities (e.g. normalisation of PR interval and QRS duration). For any patient receiving calcium or vitamin D supplements, check serum calcium levels at regular intervals or if they develop symptoms of hypercalcaemia.
Cost	Oral calcium and vitamin D preparations are relatively inexpensive on an individual patient basis, but at a population level they account for substantial healthcare spending. Calcium gluconate is inexpensive.

Clinical tip—Hyperkalaemia is common among hospital inpatients and is potentially life threatening. Calcium gluconate is the first-line emergency treatment for severe hyperkalaemia associated with ECG abnormalities. As such, you should know its dose by heart (10 mL of calcium gluconate 10% IV over 5–10 minutes).

Calcium channel blockers

CLINICAL PHARMACOLOGY

Common indications	❶ Amlodipine and, to a lesser extent, nifedipine are used for the first- or second-line treatment of **hypertension,** to reduce the risk of stroke, myocardial infarction and death from cardiovascular disease. ❷ All calcium channel blockers can be used to control symptoms in people with **stable angina;** β-blockers are the main alternative. ❸ Diltiazem and verapamil are used to control cardiac rate in people with **supraventricular arrhythmias** including supraventricular tachycardia, atrial flutter and atrial fibrillation.
Mechanisms of action	Calcium channel blockers decrease Ca^{2+} entry into vascular and cardiac cells, reducing intracellular calcium concentration. This causes **relaxation and vasodilation in arterial smooth muscle,** lowering arterial pressure. In the heart, calcium channel blockers **reduce myocardial contractility.** They **suppress cardiac conduction,** particularly across the atrioventricular (AV) node, slowing ventricular rate. Reduced cardiac rate, contractility and afterload reduce **myocardial oxygen demand,** preventing angina. Calcium channel blockers can broadly be divided into two classes. *Dihydropyridines*, including amlodipine and nifedipine, are relatively selective for the vasculature, whereas *non-dihydropyridines* are more selective for the heart. Of the *non-dihydropyridines*, verapamil is the most cardioselective, whereas diltiazem also has some effects on the vessels.
Important adverse effects	Common adverse effects of *amlodipine* and *nifedipine* include **ankle swelling, flushing, headache** and **palpitations,** which are caused by vasodilatation and compensatory tachycardia. *Verapamil* commonly causes **constipation** and less often, but more seriously, can cause **bradycardia, heart block** and **cardiac failure.** As *diltiazem* has mixed vascular and cardiac actions, it can cause any of these adverse effects.
Warnings	*Verapamil* and *diltiazem* should be used with caution in patients with ▲**poor left ventricular function** as they can precipitate or worsen heart failure. They should generally be avoided in people with ▲**AV nodal conduction delay** in whom they may provoke complete heart block. *Amlodipine* and *nifedipine* should be avoided in patients with ✖**unstable angina** as vasodilatation causes a reflex increase in contractility and tachycardia, which increases myocardial oxygen demand. In patients with ✖**severe aortic stenosis,** amlodipine and nifedipine should be avoided as they can provoke collapse.
Important interactions	Non-dihydropyridine calcium channel blockers (*verapamil* and *diltiazem)* should not be prescribed with ✖β-blockers except under close specialist supervision. Both drug classes are negatively inotropic and chronotropic, and together may cause heart failure, bradycardia, and even asystole.

amlodipine, nifedipine, diltiazem, verapamil

PRACTICAL PRESCRIBING

Prescription	Calcium channel blockers are generally taken orally; of the examples in this book, only verapamil is available for IV administration in the acute management of arrhythmias. Amlodipine has a plasma half-life of 35–50 hours and is suitable for once daily administration. By contrast, the half-lives of nifedipine (2–3 hours), verapamil (2–8 hours) and diltiazem (6–8 hours) are relatively short. Diltiazem and nifedipine are available in standard-release preparations that are taken 8-hrly, and modified-release (MR) preparations taken 12-hrly or daily. These may need to be prescribed by brand name (see Clinical tip). Example treatment regimens are: for **hypertension,** amlodipine 5–10 mg orally daily; for **angina,** diltiazem MR 90 mg orally 12-hrly; and for **supraventricular arrhythmias,** verapamil 40–120 mg orally 8-hrly.
Administration	Modified-release and long-acting preparations should be **swallowed whole,** and not crushed or chewed as this will interfere with the slow release of the drug.
Communication	Explain why the calcium channel blocker has been prescribed depending on indication. As appropriate, discuss other measures to **reduce cardiovascular risk,** including smoking cessation. Discuss **common side effects,** particularly ankle oedema if relevant.
Monitoring	Treatment efficacy can be judged by regular blood pressure monitoring for hypertension, enquiry about chest pain for angina and by pulse rate from examination or ECG. A 24-hour tape can be performed to review arrhythmias.
Cost	Amlodipine is available in non-proprietary form and is inexpensive. For diltiazem and nifedipine, only the longer-acting preparations are licensed to treat hypertension. These are more expensive.

Clinical tip—The different longer-acting preparations of nifedipine and diltiazem may not be 'bioequivalent' (i.e. pharmaceutically interchangeable). You should therefore request a specific brand when prescribing either of these drugs.

Carbamazepine

CLINICAL PHARMACOLOGY

Common indications	❶ **Epilepsy,** as a first choice treatment for focal seizures with and without secondary generalisation and for primary generalised seizures. ❷ **Trigeminal neuralgia,** as first choice treatment to control pain and reduce frequency and severity of attacks. ❸ **Bipolar disorder,** as an option for prophylaxis in patients resistant to or intolerant of other medication.
Mechanisms of action	The mechanism of action of carbamazepine is incompletely understood. It appears to **inhibit neuronal sodium channels,** stabilising resting membrane potentials and reducing neuronal excitability (see Phenytoin). This may inhibit spread of seizure activity in epilepsy, control neuralgic pain by blocking synaptic transmission in the trigeminal nucleus and stabilise mood in bipolar disorder by reducing electrical 'kindling' in the temporal lobe and limbic system.
Important adverse effects	The most common dose-related adverse effects are **gastrointestinal upset** (e.g. nausea and vomiting) and **neurological effects** (particularly dizziness and ataxia). Carbamazepine **hypersensitivity** affects about 10% of people taking the drug and most commonly manifests as a mild maculopapular skin rash. **Antiepileptic hypersensitivity syndrome** affects about 1 in 5000 people taking carbamazepine or phenytoin, usually within 2 months of starting treatment. Clinical features include severe skin reactions (e.g. Stevens–Johnson syndrome, toxic epidermal necrolysis), fever and lymphadenopathy with systemic (e.g. haematological, hepatic, renal) involvement and mortality of about 10%. Other common adverse effects include **oedema** and **hyponatraemia** due to an antidiuretic hormone-like effect.
Warnings	Carbamazepine exposure *in utero* is associated with neural tube defects, cardiac and urinary tract abnormalities and cleft palate. Women with epilepsy planning ▲**pregnancy** should discuss treatment with a specialist and start taking high-dose folic acid supplements before conception. Prior ✖**antiepileptic hypersensitivity syndrome** is a contraindication to both carbamazepine and phenytoin, due to potential cross-sensitivity. Carbamazepine should be prescribed with caution in patients with ▲**hepatic, renal or cardiac disease,** due to increased risk of toxicity.
Important interactions	Carbamazepine induces cytochrome P450 enzymes, reducing plasma concentration and efficacy of ▲**drugs that are metabolised by P450 enzymes** (e.g. warfarin, oestrogens and progestogens). Carbamazepine is itself metabolised by these enzymes, so its concentration and adverse effects are increased by ▲**cytochrome P450 inhibitors** (e.g. macrolides). Complex interactions occur with ▲**other antiepileptic drugs** as most alter drug metabolism. The efficacy of antiepileptic drugs is reduced by ▲**drugs that lower the seizure threshold** (e.g. SSRIs, tricyclic antidepressants, antipsychotics, tramadol).

PRACTICAL PRESCRIBING

Prescription	Carbamazepine is only available for oral or rectal administration. It is usually **started at a low dose,** e.g. 100–200 mg once or twice daily to limit dose-related adverse effects. As tolerance develops to adverse effects, the dose is **increased gradually** to a usual maximum of 1.6 g/day in divided doses. Treatment should not be stopped suddenly, but should be withdrawn gradually under medical supervision, due to risk of seizure recurrence.
Administration	Oral carbamazepine is available as immediate- or modified-release tablets, chewable tablets and oral suspension. As carbamazepine bioavailability differs between formulations, ▲switching between them is best avoided. Use of rectal suppositories should be limited to short periods when oral administration is not possible as rectal irritation may occur with prolonged use.
Communication	Explain that treatment aims to reduce seizure frequency. Warn the patient to look out for signs of severe hypersensitivity, including skin rashes; bruising, bleeding, a high temperature or mouth ulcers (blood toxicity); reduced appetite or abdominal pain (liver toxicity). If any of these occur they should seek urgent medical advice. For women, discuss contraception and pregnancy (see Valproate). Advise patients that they must not drive unless they have been seizure-free for 12 months (or have at least a three-year pattern of seizures while asleep only). They should not drive for 6 months after changing or stopping treatment.
Monitoring	Treatment **efficacy** is monitored by comparing seizure frequency before and after starting treatment or dose adjustment. The most useful way to monitor **safety** is by asking the patient to report any unusual symptoms immediately (as above). Routine measurement of full blood count and liver enzymes is unlikely to coincide with unpredictable hypersensitivity reactions. **Plasma carbamazepine concentrations** are not routinely measured, but may be useful in selected cases. Blood should be taken immediately before the next dose, when carbamazepine concentrations should be 4–12 mg/L. Time to steady-state plasma concentrations (and appropriate sampling for repeat measurements) is 2–4 weeks after starting treatment and 4–5 days after a dose change.
Cost	Carbamazepine in any formulation is inexpensive.

Clinical tip—Newer antiepileptic drugs (e.g. lamotrigine, levetiracetam [Keppra®]) are increasingly used. There is no evidence that they are more effective than older drugs but they may be better tolerated. Initial choice of antiepileptic drug should be based on seizure type, epilepsy syndrome, co-medication, comorbidities and patient choice. Carbamazepine is usually the first choice for focal seizures.

Cephalosporins and carbapenems

CLINICAL PHARMACOLOGY

Common indications	❶ Oral cephalosporins are second- and third-line treatment options for **urinary** and **respiratory tract infections.** ❷ Intravenous cephalosporins and carbapenems are reserved for the treatment of infections that are **very severe** or **complicated,** or caused by **antibiotic-resistant organisms.** Due to their broad antimicrobial spectrum they can be used for most indications (with these caveats).
Mechanisms of action	Cephalosporins and carbapenems are derived from naturally occurring antimicrobials produced by fungi and bacteria. Like <u>penicillins</u>, their antimicrobial effect is due to their **β-lactam ring.** During bacterial cell growth, cephalosporins and carbapenems inhibit enzymes responsible for cross-linking peptidoglycans in bacterial cell walls. This weakens cell walls, preventing them from maintaining an osmotic gradient, resulting in **bacterial cell swelling, lysis** and **death.** Both types of antibiotic have a **broad spectrum of action.** For cephalosporins, progressive structural modification has led to successive 'generations' (first to fifth), with increasing activity against Gram-negative bacteria and less oral activity. Cephalosporins and carbapenems are naturally more **resistant to β-lactamases** than penicillins due to fusion of the β-lactam ring with a dihydrothiazine ring (*cephalosporins*) or a unique hydroxyethyl side chain (*carbapenems*).
Important adverse effects	**Gastrointestinal upset,** such as nausea and diarrhoea, are common. Less frequently, **antibiotic-associated colitis** occurs when broad-spectrum antibiotics kill normal gut flora, allowing overgrowth of toxin-producing *Clostridium difficile.* This is debilitating and can be complicated by colonic perforation and death. **Hypersensitivity,** including immediate and delayed reactions may occur (see <u>Penicillins</u>). As cephalosporins and carbapenem share structural similarities to penicillins, cross-reactivity may occur with some penicillin-allergic patients. There is a risk of **central nervous system toxicity** including **seizures,** particularly where carbapenems are prescribed in high dose or to patients with renal impairment.
Warnings	Cephalosporins and carbapenems should be used with caution in people **at risk of *C. difficile* infection,** particularly those in hospital and the elderly. The main contraindication is history of ▲**allergy** to a penicillin, cephalosporin or carbapenem, particularly if there was an ✖**anaphylactic reaction.** *Carbapenems* should be used with caution in patients with ▲**epilepsy.** A dose reduction is required for both drug classes in ▲**renal impairment.**
Important interactions	As broad-spectrum antibiotics, cephalosporins and carbapenems can enhance the anticoagulant effect of <u>warfarin</u> by killing normal gut flora that synthesise vitamin K. Cephalosporins may increase nephrotoxicity of <u>aminoglycosides</u>. Carbapenems reduce plasma concentration and efficacy of <u>valproate</u>.

cefalexin, cefotaxime, meropenem, ertapenem

PRACTICAL PRESCRIBING

Prescription	*Cephalosporins* are usually prescribed for 6–12-hrly administration. Only certain cephalosporins (e.g. cefalexin) are orally active. Intravenous cephalosporins are used at high dose for severe infections (e.g. cefotaxime 2 g IV 6-hrly for bacterial meningitis). *Carbapenems* are only available for IV administration (e.g. meropenem 1–2 g IV 8-hrly).
Administration	*Cephalosporins* can be administered orally, as tablets, capsules or oral suspension, or by injection, which can be IV, as bolus injection or infusion, or IM. *Carbapenems* can be administered as IV injection or infusion. Ertapenem is a carbapenem that is administered once daily. This facilitates outpatient administration of IV antibiotic therapy and allows patients needing prolonged treatment to be at home.
Communication	Explain that the aim of treatment is to get rid of infection and improve symptoms. For oral treatment, encourage the patient to complete the prescribed course. Before prescribing, always check with your patient personally or get collateral history to ensure they do not have an **allergy** to any form of penicillin or other β-lactam antibiotics. Warn them to seek medical advice if a rash or other unexpected symptoms develop. If an allergy develops during treatment, give the patient written and verbal advice not to take this antibiotic in the future and make sure that the allergy is clearly documented in their medical records.
Monitoring	Check that infection resolves by symptoms, signs (e.g. resolution of pyrexia) and blood tests (e.g. falling C-reactive protein and white cell count).
Cost	The costs of IV antibiotic therapy include drugs, administration time and equipment, complications (e.g. *C. difficile* infection), and need for inpatient stay. Where clinically appropriate, costs can be reduced by limiting duration of antibiotic therapy, IV-to-oral antibiotic switch during recovery and outpatient administration of IV antibiotics.

Clinical tip—Individual hospitals have antibiotic policies to protect valuable antibiotics from the development of resistance and reduce the risk of hospital-acquired infection. In many hospitals, intravenous cephalosporins and carbapenems can only be prescribed with the approval of a microbiologist. As antibiotic-associated colitis seems to occur more commonly with second and third generation cephalosporins, their use is now particularly restricted. Always get to know and follow your local antibiotic guidelines and seek microbiology advice where these do not cover a specific clinical situation.

Clopidogrel

CLINICAL PHARMACOLOGY

Common indications	Clopidogrel is generally prescribed with <u>aspirin</u>, although clopidogrel may be used alone where aspirin is contraindicated or not tolerated. ❶ For treatment of **acute coronary syndrome** (ACS), where rapid inhibition of platelet aggregation can prevent or limit arterial thrombosis and reduce subsequent mortality. ❷ To prevent occlusion of **coronary artery stents.** ❸ For long-term secondary prevention of thrombotic arterial events in patients with **cardiovascular, cerebrovascular and peripheral arterial disease.** ❹ To reduce the risk of intracardiac thrombus and embolic stroke in **atrial fibrillation** where <u>warfarin</u> and novel oral anticoagulants are contraindicated.
Mechanisms of action	Thrombotic events occur when platelet-rich thrombus forms in atheromatous arteries and occludes the circulation. Clopidogrel **prevents platelet aggregation** and reduces the risk of arterial occlusion by binding irreversibly to **adenosine diphosphate (ADP) receptors** (P2Y$_{12}$ subtype) on the surface of platelets. As this process is independent of the cyclooxygenase pathway, its actions are synergistic with those of aspirin.
Important adverse effects	The most common adverse effect of clopidogrel is **bleeding,** which can be serious, particularly if gastrointestinal, intracranial or following a surgical procedure. **Gastrointestinal upset,** including dyspepsia, abdominal pain and diarrhoea, is also common. As with other antiplatelet agents, clopidogrel can rarely affect platelet numbers as well as function, causing **thrombocytopenia.**
Warnings	Clopidogrel should not be prescribed for people with significant ✖**active bleeding** and may need to be stopped 7 days before ▲**elective surgery** and other procedures (see Clinical tip). It should be used with caution in patients with ▲**renal and hepatic impairment,** especially where patients otherwise have an increased risk of bleeding.
Important interactions	Clopidogrel is a **pro-drug** that requires metabolism by hepatic cytochrome P450 enzymes to its active form to have antiplatelet effect. Its efficacy may be reduced by ▲**cytochrome P450 inhibitors** by *inhibiting its activation.* Relevant examples include <u>omeprazole</u>, <u>ciprofloxacin</u>, <u>erythromycin</u>, some <u>antifungals</u> and some <u>SSRIs</u>. Where gastroprotection with a proton pump inhibitor (see Aspirin) is required for patients taking clopidogrel, <u>lansoprazole</u> or <u>pantoprazole</u> are preferred over omeprazole as they are considered less likely to inhibit clopidogrel activation. Co-prescription of clopidogrel with other ▲**antiplatelet drugs** (e.g. <u>aspirin</u>), ▲**anticoagulants** (e.g. <u>heparin</u>) or ▲NSAIDs increases the risk of bleeding.

PRACTICAL PRESCRIBING

Prescription	Clopidogrel is only available as an oral preparation. Low doses of clopidogrel require up to a week to reach their full antiplatelet effect. When rapid effect is needed you should prescribe a **loading dose,** normally 300 mg orally for ACS, in the once-only section of the drug chart before commencing a regular **maintenance dose** of 75 mg orally daily. It is good practice to write the indication and intended duration of antiplatelet therapy as additional instructions on the inpatient and discharge prescriptions. This is of particular importance following the insertion of a **drug-eluting coronary stent.** In this context, dual antiplatelet therapy should be continued for **12 months** to reduce the risk of stent thrombosis and should not be discontinued prematurely without prior discussion with a cardiologist.
Administration	Clopidogrel can be given with or without food.
Communication	Advise patients that the purpose of treatment is to reduce the risk of heart attacks or strokes and to prolong life. In those who are taking clopidogrel following the insertion of a drug-eluting stent, emphasise the importance of continuing treatment as directed, usually for 12 months, to make sure that the stent stays open and does not block and cause a heart attack. Before starting therapy, check that the patient does not have any active bleeding. Explain that if bleeding does occur while on treatment it might take longer than usual to stop. Patients should report any unusual or sustained bleeding to their doctor.
Monitoring	Clinical monitoring for adverse effects is most appropriate.
Cost	Clopidogrel is available as an inexpensive non-proprietary preparation.

Clinical tip—Clopidogrel acts irreversibly. It therefore takes the lifespan of a platelet (around 7 to 10 days) for its antiplatelet effect to wear off. Clopidogrel should be stopped 7 days before elective surgery or other invasive procedures, unless the risk of stopping clopidogrel exceeds the risk of continuing. Thus in patients who have had a drug-eluting coronary artery stent inserted within the last 12 months, surgery should be delayed if possible. In emergency cases, patients taking clopidogrel may require platelet infusion to help stop bleeding.

Compound (β₂-agonist–corticosteroid) inhalers

CLINICAL PHARMACOLOGY

Common indications	❶ **Asthma:** control of symptoms and prevention of exacerbations, used at 'steps 3–4' in the management of chronic asthma. ❷ **Chronic obstructive pulmonary disease (COPD):** to control symptoms and prevent exacerbations in patients who have severe airflow obstruction on spirometry and/or recurrent exacerbations.
Mechanisms of action	Compound inhalers contain an inhaled corticosteroid to suppress airway inflammation, and a long-acting β₂-agonist (LABA) to stimulate bronchodilation. The prescription of these drugs in combination reduces the number of different inhalers that need to be taken and increases adherence to treatment. In **asthma,** compound inhalers ensure that long-acting β₂-agonists are not taken without an inhaled corticosteroid. This is important because, without a steroid, long-acting β₂-agonists are associated with increased asthma deaths. In **COPD,** combined treatment is more effective in reducing exacerbations than either drug alone. Seretide® contains fluticasone and salmeterol. Symbicort® contains budesonide and formoterol.
Important adverse effects	*Inhaled corticosteroids* most commonly cause local adverse effects, including **oral thrush** and a **hoarse voice.** There is some evidence that they increase the risk of **pneumonia** in people with COPD. Where used at very high doses for a long time, **systemic adverse effects** including adrenal suppression, growth retardation (children) and osteoporosis may occur. *Long-acting β₂-agonists* can cause **tremor, tachycardia, arrhythmias** and **muscle cramps.**
Warnings	High-dose *inhaled corticosteroids*, particularly fluticasone, should be used with caution in ▲**COPD patients with a history of pneumonia** and in ▲**children,** where there is potential for growth suppression. Care should be taken when prescribing *long-acting β₂-agonists* for patients with ▲**cardiovascular disease,** in whom tachycardia may provoke angina or arrhythmias.
Important interactions	Interactions are not generally a problem due to low systemic absorption. However β-blockers may reduce the effectiveness of β₂-agonists.

PRACTICAL PRESCRIBING

Prescription	You should prescribe compound inhalers by proprietary (brand) name, inhaler type and strength. Strength describes the amount of medicine per inhalation, e.g. Symbicort® Turbohaler 400/12 contains 400 micrograms of budesonide and 12 micrograms of formoterol per inhalation. Seretide® 500 Accuhaler contains fluticasone 500 micrograms and salmeterol 50 micrograms per inhalation. You should specify the number of inhalations and dosing frequency, e.g. Symbicort Turbohaler® 400/12 two puffs twice daily.
Administration	Seretide® is formulated as pressurised metered dose (Evohaler) and dry powder (Accuhaler) inhalers. Symbicort® is available as a dry powder inhaler (Turbohaler). Provision of a spacer with metered dose inhalers can improve airway deposition and treatment efficacy and reduce oral adverse effects. The patient should be trained how to use their inhaler and technique should be checked and corrected at every consultation.
Communication	You should advise your patient that this new inhaler will help prevent attacks and improve breathlessness, but **must be taken without fail** every morning and evening to have this benefit. You should emphasise that they may not notice immediate benefit from the inhaler, but that an improvement should be felt over hours and days. You should reassure them that inhaled steroids generally **do not cause whole-body side effects** (e.g. weight gain). Advise them to **rinse their mouth and gargle** after taking the inhaler to prevent development of a sore mouth or hoarse voice. Show your patient how to use the device and check and correct their technique as necessary every time you see them.
Monitoring	You should check if the treatment has worked by asking the patient about symptoms and reviewing peak flow measurements (asthma) or exacerbation frequency (COPD and asthma). You should enquire about adverse effects, particularly sore mouth or change in voice.
Cost	Compound inhalers account for a large slice of the NHS drugs budget. Costs can be reduced by ensuring the inhaler is only prescribed if indicated, is stopped if ineffective and that the cheapest formulation available is prescribed.

Clinical tip—The long-acting bronchodilator formoterol (in Symbicort®) has a relatively quick onset of action, so can be used as both a short- and long-acting reliever, which can simplify treatment for patients with asthma (SMART regimen). Formoterol dosage is more flexible (6–36 micrograms twice daily) than salmeterol dosage (50 micrograms twice daily), making it easier to step asthma treatment up and down with Symbicort® than Seretide®. However, fluticasone (in Seretide®) is more potent than budesonide (in Symbicort®) so may be more effective in severe asthma.

Corticosteroids (glucocorticoids), systemic

CLINICAL PHARMACOLOGY

Common indications	❶ To treat **allergic** or **inflammatory disorders,** e.g. anaphylaxis, asthma. ❷ Suppression of **autoimmune disease,** e.g. inflammatory bowel disease, inflammatory arthritis. ❸ In the treatment of some **cancers** as part of chemotherapy or to reduce tumour-associated swelling. ❹ Hormone replacement in **adrenal insufficiency** or **hypopituitarism.**
Mechanisms of action	These corticosteroids exert mainly glucocorticoid effects. They bind to cytosolic glucocorticoid receptors, which then translocate to the nucleus and bind to glucocorticoid-response elements, which regulate gene expression. Corticosteroids are most commonly prescribed to **modify the immune response**. They **upregulate anti-inflammatory genes** and **downregulate pro-inflammatory genes** (e.g. cytokines, tumour necrosis factor alpha). Direct actions on inflammatory cells include suppression of circulating monocytes and eosinophils. Their **metabolic effects** include increased gluconeogenesis from increased circulating amino and fatty acids, released by catabolism (breakdown) of muscle and fat. These drugs also have **mineralocorticoid effects**, stimulating Na^+ and water retention and K^+ excretion in the renal tubule.
Important adverse effects	**Immunosuppression** increases the risk and severity of infection and alters the host response. **Metabolic** effects include diabetes mellitus and osteoporosis. Increased catabolism causes proximal muscle weakness, skin thinning with easy bruising and gastritis. **Mood** and **behavioural changes** include insomnia, confusion, psychosis and suicidal ideas. Hypertension, hypokalaemia and oedema can result from **mineralocorticoid** actions. Corticosteroid treatment suppresses pituitary adrenocorticotropic hormone (ACTH) secretion, switching off the stimulus for normal adrenal cortisol production. In *prolonged treatment*, this causes **adrenal atrophy,** preventing endogenous cortisol secretion. If corticosteroids are withdrawn suddenly, an acute **Addisonian crisis** with cardiovascular collapse may occur. Slow withdrawal is required to allow recovery of adrenal function. Symptoms of **chronic glucocorticoid deficiency** that occur during treatment withdrawal include fatigue, weight loss and arthralgia.
Warnings	Corticosteroids should be prescribed with caution in people with ▲**infection** and in ▲**children** (in whom they can suppress growth).
Important interactions	Corticosteroids increase the risk of peptic ulceration and gastrointestinal bleeding when used with <u>NSAIDs</u> and enhance hypokalaemia in patients taking β_2-agonists, theophylline, <u>loop</u> or <u>thiazide diuretics</u>. Their efficacy may be reduced by ▲**cytochrome P450 inducers** (e.g. <u>phenytoin</u>, <u>carbamazepine</u>, rifampicin). Corticosteroids reduce the immune response to <u>vaccines</u>.

prednisolone, hydrocortisone, dexamethasone

PRACTICAL PRESCRIBING

Prescription	Different corticosteroids have different anti-inflammatory potencies. Of the examples given, dexamethasone is the most potent, with a dose of 750 micrograms being equivalent to prednisolone 5 mg and hydrocortisone 20 mg. Systemic corticosteroid treatment can be given orally or by IV or IM injection. In emergencies (e.g. treatment of **cerebral oedema caused by cancer**), dexamethasone is prescribed at a high dose (e.g. 8 mg twice daily orally or IV), then weaned slowly as symptoms improve. In acute asthma, prednisolone is usually prescribed at a dose of 40 mg orally daily. Where oral administration is inappropriate (e.g. **inflammatory bowel disease flares, anaphylaxis**), IV hydrocortisone may be used. In long-term treatment, e.g. for **inflammatory arthritis,** use the lowest dose of oral prednisolone that controls disease while limiting adverse effects. This may require co-prescription of steroid-sparing agents (e.g. azathioprine, methotrexate). Also consider the use of bisphosphonates and proton pump inhibitors to reduce some of the steroid side effects.
Administration	Once daily corticosteroid treatment should be taken in the morning, to mimic the natural circadian rhythm and reduce insomnia.
Communication	Explain that treatment should suppress the underlying disease process and that the patient will usually **start to feel better within 1–2 days.** For patients who require prolonged treatment, warn them **not to stop treatment suddenly,** as this could make them very unwell. Give them a steroid card to carry with them at all times and show if they need treatment. Discuss the benefits and risks of steroids, including longer-term risks of osteoporosis, bone fractures and diabetes so that your patient can make an informed decision about taking treatment.
Monitoring	Monitoring of **efficacy** will depend on the condition treated, e.g. peak flow recordings for asthma, blood inflammatory markers for inflammatory arthritis. In prolonged treatment, monitor for **adverse effects** by, for example, measuring glucose and HbA_{1c} or performing a dual-energy X-ray absorptiometry (DEXA) scan to look for osteoporosis.
Cost	Prednisolone, hydrocortisone and dexamethasone are all available in non-proprietary form and are inexpensive.

Clinical tip—Patients on long-term corticosteroid therapy have atrophic adrenal glands and may be unable to increase cortisol secretion in response to stress. You may therefore need to provide this artificially by increasing the dose of exogenous corticosteroid. Common practice is to double the dose during acute illness, reducing back to the maintenance dose on recovery.

Corticosteroids (glucocorticoids), inhaled

CLINICAL PHARMACOLOGY

Common indications	❶ **Asthma:** to treat airways inflammation and control symptoms at 'step 2' of therapy where asthma is not adequately controlled by a short-acting β₂-agonist alone. ❷ **Chronic obstructive pulmonary disease (COPD):** to control symptoms and prevent exacerbations in patients who have severe airflow obstruction on spirometry and/or recurrent exacerbations. Inhaled corticosteroids are usually prescribed in combination with a long-acting β₂-agonist and/or a long-acting antimuscarinic bronchodilator.
Mechanisms of action	Corticosteroids pass through the plasma membrane and interact with receptors in the cytoplasm. The activated receptor then passes into the nucleus to modify the transcription of a large number of genes. Pro-inflammatory interleukins, cytokines and chemokines are downregulated, while anti-inflammatory proteins are upregulated. In the airways, **this reduces mucosal inflammation, widens the airways, and reduces mucus** secretion. This **improves symptoms and reduces exacerbations** in asthma and COPD.
Important adverse effects	The main adverse effects of inhaled corticosteroids occur locally in the airway, where their immunosuppressive effect can cause **oral candidiasis** (thrush infection). They can also cause a **hoarse voice.** In COPD, there is some evidence they may increase the risk of **pneumonia.** Very little is absorbed into the blood, so there are few systemic adverse effects unless taken at very high dose when systemic side effects including adrenal suppression, growth retardation (children) and osteoporosis may occur.
Warnings	High-dose inhaled corticosteroids, particularly fluticasone, should be used with caution in COPD patients with a ▲**history of pneumonia** and in ▲**children,** where there is potential for growth suppression.
Important interactions	There are no clinically significant adverse drug interactions with inhaled corticosteroids.

beclometasone, budesonide, fluticasone

PRACTICAL PRESCRIBING

Prescription	A variety of inhaler devices are available. Selecting the device that best suits the patient is important, and this may dictate drug choice. Inhaled corticosteroids should usually be prescribed for **twice daily administration,** with dose depending on the drug chosen and severity of illness. For example, beclometasone (e.g. as Clenil Modulite® metered dose inhaler) 100 micrograms, two puffs twice daily would be an option for step 2 treatment of asthma. Brand name prescribing may be necessary as different preparations of the same drug may have different potencies depending on how they are deposited in the airway.
Administration	Drugs are delivered in **aerosol** (metered dose inhaler [MDI]) or **dry powder** form. Provision of a **spacer with metered dose inhalers** can improve airway deposition and treatment efficacy and reduce oral adverse effects. The patient should be trained how to use their **inhaler** and **technique** should be checked and corrected at every consultation.
Communication	Explain that you are offering a steroid inhaler to 'dampen down' inflammation in the lung. Reassure them that hardly any of the steroid is absorbed into the body so, except in very high-dose treatment, there are unlikely to be any serious side effects (or weight gain). Advise them to rinse their mouth and gargle after taking the inhaler to prevent development of a sore mouth or hoarse voice. Show your patient how to use the device and check and correct their technique as necessary every time you see them.
Monitoring	Patients with asthma can monitor their disease severity through symptoms and serial peak expiratory flow rate measurements. They may be able to adjust their own treatment with guidance from a written 'action plan.' Likewise, symptom severity and exacerbation rates are the main indicators of effect in COPD. In general, a review after 3–6 months of therapy should be undertaken to see if therapy should be maintained or stepped up or down.
Cost	In general, inhalers that contain corticosteroids only are relatively cheap, whereas combination inhalers are more expensive.

Clinical tip—Poorly controlled airway inflammation in asthma can lead to airways remodelling and fixed airflow obstruction. As inflammation is generally steroid-responsive, patients with **asthma** should be strongly encouraged to **take sufficient inhaled corticosteroids to control symptoms and prevent disease progression.** By contrast, airways inflammation in COPD is poorly responsive to steroids and, although inhaled corticosteroids can improve lung function and reduce exacerbations, they do not prevent disease progression.

Corticosteroids (glucocorticoids), topical

CLINICAL PHARMACOLOGY

Common indications	❶ Used in inflammatory skin conditions, e.g. **eczema,** to treat disease flares or to control chronic disease where <u>emollients</u> alone are ineffective.
Mechanisms of action	Corticosteroids have **immunosuppressive, metabolic** and **mineralocorticoid** effects, as discussed in detail under <u>Corticosteroids (glucocorticoids), systemic</u>. Where corticosteroids are applied topically, effects are mostly limited to the site of application. With potent or prolonged use of topical corticosteroids, systemic absorption and effects can occur. Topical corticosteroids can be classified as being mild, moderately potent, potent and very potent, depending on the type and concentration of corticosteroid in the formulation. Of the examples given, hydrocortisone 0.1–2.5% is mild and betamethasone valerate 0.1% is potent.
Important adverse effects	Adverse effects are uncommon with mild or moderately potent topical corticosteroids. However, potent and very potent topical corticosteroids can cause **local adverse effects** such as skin thinning, striae, telangiectasia and contact dermatitis. When used on the face, they can cause perioral dermatitis and cause or exacerbate acne. Withdrawal of topical corticosteroids can cause a **rebound worsening** of the underlying skin condition. Rarely, **adrenal suppression** and **systemic adverse effects** occur (see <u>Corticosteroids (glucocorticoids), systemic</u>).
Warnings	You should not use topical corticosteroids where ▲**infection** is present as this can cause the infection to worsen or spread. Where ▲**facial lesions** are present, potent corticosteroids should be avoided and treatment courses should be short.
Important interactions	There are generally no significant drug interactions when corticosteroids are used topically. If several topical agents are being used on the same area of skin, applications should be spaced out to allow absorption of pharmacologically active agents; <u>emollients</u> should be applied last.

hydrocortisone, betamethasone

PRACTICAL PRESCRIBING

Prescription	General advice when prescribing topical corticosteroids is to use as mild a corticosteroid as possible for as short a time as possible, usually for no more than 2 weeks (1 week for facial lesions). When prescribing for **eczema,** choose mild corticosteroids for mild flares, moderately potent corticosteroids for moderate flares and potent corticosteroids for severe flares. Indicate the potency of the steroid alongside its name as part of the prescription. Your prescription should state the name and strength of the corticosteroid, the formulation required (e.g. lotion, cream, ointment [see Emollients]), and the amount to be supplied, e.g. *hydrocortisone 1% (mild) cream, supply 30 g*. Note that the strength of hydrocortisone is expressed as a percentage (1%), which indicates the number of grams of drug (1 g) in 100 g of cream. You also need to define the area of skin that the corticosteroid should be applied to and state that it should be applied one to two times daily. The amount to be supplied will depend on the area of skin to be covered. For example 30–60 g of cream or ointment should cover both arms for a 2 week course.
Administration	Corticosteroids should be **applied very thinly** and **only to the area of skin where disease is active.** You may find that creams are easier to apply to moist lesions, while ointments are more suitable where skin has become thick and leathery (lichenified). Wash hands after application (unless they are being treated!).
Communication	Explain that you are providing a therapy that will relieve inflammation and improve their skin problem, but that the full effect may take 1–2 weeks. Inform them how and when to apply the topical corticosteroid and that emollients should be applied 5 minutes after this. **Warn them of the risk of skin damage if the treatment is applied to the wrong areas or for too long.** The pharmacist should make sure that the instructions are stuck directly onto the tube of cream or ointment and not onto the outside packaging, which may be discarded.
Monitoring	Review the patient after 1–2 weeks of treatment to ensure that symptoms are improving and treatment instructions are being followed correctly.
Cost	All topical corticosteroids are relatively inexpensive. Mild topical corticosteroids can be purchased over the counter with advice from a pharmacist.

Clinical tip—Explaining how to apply the correct amount of topical corticosteroids can be tricky. The BNF advises that if a length of cream or ointment is squeezed from its tube to run from the fingertip to the first crease of an adult finger, this should provide enough cream or ointment to cover an area of skin approximately twice the size of the palm.

Digoxin

CLINICAL PHARMACOLOGY

Common indications	❶ In **atrial fibrillation (AF)** and **atrial flutter,** digoxin is used to reduce the ventricular rate. However, a β-blocker or non-dihydropyridine calcium channel blocker is usually more effective. ❷ In **severe heart failure,** digoxin is used as a third-line treatment in patients who are already taking an ACE inhibitor, β-blocker and either an aldosterone antagonist or angiotensin receptor blocker. It is used at an earlier stage in patients with co-existing AF.
Mechanisms of action	Digoxin is **negatively chronotropic** (it reduces the heart rate) and **positively inotropic** (it increases the force of contraction). In **atrial fibrillation and flutter** its therapeutic effect arises mainly via an indirect pathway involving increased vagal (parasympathetic) tone. This reduces conduction at the atrioventricular (AV) node, preventing some impulses from being transmitted to the ventricles, thereby reducing the ventricular rate. In **heart failure,** it has a direct effect on myocytes through inhibition of Na^+/K^+-ATPase pumps, causing Na^+ to accumulate in the cell. As cellular extrusion of Ca^{2+} requires low intracellular Na^+ concentrations, elevation of intracellular Na^+ causes Ca^{2+} to accumulate in the cell, increasing contractile force.
Important adverse effects	Adverse effects of digoxin include **bradycardia, gastrointestinal disturbance, rash, dizziness** and **visual disturbance** (blurred or yellow vision). Digoxin is proarrhythmic and has a low therapeutic index: that is, the safety margin between the therapeutic and toxic doses is narrow. A wide range of arrhythmias can occur in **digoxin toxicity** and these may be life threatening.
Warnings	Digoxin may worsen conduction abnormalities, so is contraindicated in ✖**second-degree heart block** and ✖**intermittent complete heart block.** It should not be used in patients with or at risk of ✖**ventricular arrhythmias.** The dose should be reduced in ▲**renal failure,** as digoxin is eliminated by the kidneys. Certain electrolyte abnormalities increase the risk of digoxin toxicity, including ▲**hypokalaemia,** ▲**hypomagnesaemia** and ▲**hypercalcaemia.** Potassium disturbance is probably the most important of these, as digoxin competes with potassium to bind the Na^+/K^+-ATPase pump. When serum potassium levels are low, competition is reduced and the effects of digoxin are enhanced.
Important interactions	Loop and thiazide diuretics can increase the risk of digoxin toxicity by causing hypokalaemia. Amiodarone, calcium channel blockers, spironolactone and quinine can all increase the plasma concentration of digoxin and therefore risk of toxicity.

PRACTICAL PRESCRIBING

Prescription	Digoxin is available as an oral or intravenous preparation. The effect of IV digoxin is seen at about 30 minutes, compared to about 2 hours following an oral dose. Intravenous administration is therefore usually unnecessary. Due to its large volume of distribution, a **loading dose** is required if a rapid effect is needed. A common approach is to give 500 micrograms of digoxin, followed by 250–500 micrograms 6 hours later, depending on response. Thereafter, the usual maintenance dose is 125–250 micrograms daily. For hospital inpatients, the loading doses are prescribed in the once-only section of the drug chart, while the maintenance dose is prescribed in the regular section (starting on day 2). Be sure to write 'micrograms' in full.
Administration	Oral digoxin can be taken with or without food. Intravenous doses must be given slowly.
Communication	Explain that you are offering a treatment which, as applicable, should slow down their abnormally fast heart rhythm and make their heart beat more strongly. You should warn your patient of common side effects such as sickness, diarrhoea and headache. Ask them to seek advice if side effects are particularly bad or seem to get progressively worse, as this may suggest the dose is too high.
Monitoring	The best guide to the effectiveness of digoxin is the patient's **symptoms** and **heart rate.** Check their ECG, electrolytes and renal function periodically, and particularly when these may change (e.g. during acute illnesses or after a change in medication). You should note that therapeutic doses of digoxin can cause ST-segment depression (the **'reverse tick'** sign) on the ECG. This is an expected effect and does not signify toxicity. In acute therapy, continuous cardiac monitoring is advisable. You do not need to monitor digoxin levels routinely, but it may be helpful to measure these if you suspect toxicity. High plasma concentrations of digoxin do not always indicate toxicity, but the likelihood of toxicity increases as digoxin plasma concentrations increase. Conversely, toxicity can occur even when digoxin concentration is within the 'therapeutic range'.
Cost	Digoxin is available in non-proprietary form at low cost.

Clinical tip—Because digoxin's effect on ventricular rate in AF relies on parasympathetic ('rest and digest') tone, it tends to be lost during stress and exercise. Digoxin is therefore now rarely used on its own for AF, although it may be an option in sedentary patients.

Dipyridamole

CLINICAL PHARMACOLOGY

Common indications	❶ **Cerebrovascular disease** for secondary prevention of stroke. Dipyridamole is currently first-line therapy following a **transient ischaemic attack,** and second-line therapy following an **ischaemic stroke** where <u>clopidogrel</u> is contraindicated or not tolerated. It should usually be given in combination with <u>aspirin</u> but can be used as monotherapy if aspirin is contraindicated or not tolerated. ❷ To induce tachycardia during a **myocardial perfusion scan** in the diagnosis of ischaemic heart disease.
Mechanisms of action	Dipyridamole has both antiplatelet and vasodilatory effects. Although the exact mechanism of its antiplatelet action is controversial, the end effect is an increase in intra-platelet cyclic adenosine monophosphate (cAMP) that inhibits platelet aggregation, reducing the risk of arterial occlusion. Dipyridamole also blocks cellular uptake of adenosine, prolonging its effect on blood vessels to produce vasodilation.
Important adverse effects	The side effects of dipyridamole relate to its vasodilatory effects and include **headache, flushing, dizziness** and **gastrointestinal symptoms** that normally improve with time. As with other antiplatelet agents there is an **increased risk of bleeding.** Rarely dipyridamole can affect platelet numbers as well as function, causing **thrombocytopaenia.**
Warnings	Dipyridamole should be used with caution in patients with ▲**ischaemic heart disease,** ▲**aortic stenosis** and ▲**heart failure** as it causes vasodilatation and tachycardia that can exacerbate these conditions. This effect is exploited diagnostically in myocardial perfusion scans, where radionucleotide distribution is compared in heart muscle at baseline and during tachycardia induced by intravenous dipyridamole. Reduced perfusion after dipyridamole indicates cardiac ischaemia.
Important interactions	Dipyridamole inhibits cellular uptake of ▲<u>adenosine</u>. This prolongs its effects on the heart, increasing the risk of cardiac arrest. The dose of adenosine should therefore be reduced in patients treated with dipyridamole. There is an increased risk of bleeding where dipyridamole is combined with other ▲**antiplatelet agents** (<u>aspirin</u>, <u>clopidogrel</u>) and ▲**anticoagulants** (<u>heparin</u>, <u>warfarin</u>).

dipyridamole

PRACTICAL PRESCRIBING

Prescription	For therapeutic purposes, dipyridamole is given orally. Current evidence is strongest for the use of modified-release (MR) preparations in secondary prevention of stroke. For this indication you should prescribe dipyridamole MR, 200 mg twice daily. Dipyridamole is a long-term treatment that should only usually be stopped if adverse effects are intolerable or new contraindications develop.
Administration	Dipyridamole should be taken orally, preferably with food. Modified-release preparations should be swallowed whole, and not crushed or chewed as this will interfere with the slow release of the drug.
Communication	Advise patients that the purpose of dipyridamole treatment is to **reduce the risk of further strokes** and explain that they should keep taking it indefinitely. Warn them that there is an **increased risk of bleeding,** and that they should report any unusual bleeding to their doctor. Patients can be reassured that **initial side effects** such as headache, flushing, dizziness and gastrointestinal disturbances should improve with time.
Monitoring	Enquiry about side effects is the most appropriate form of monitoring.
Cost	Although dipyridamole MR is currently only available as a branded formulation and is slightly more expensive than immediate-release (IR) preparations, it should be prescribed due to superior evidence of efficacy (see Prescription).

Clinical tip—Headache is a common side effect of dipyridamole but tends to wear off over time. To minimise headache, start dipyridamole at a low dose and gradually increase this over a period of 2 weeks, e.g. 100 mg once daily for 1 week, increased to 100 mg twice daily in the second week, and then to 200 mg twice daily in the third week. As dipyridamole MR only comes as 200 mg capsules, this may require initiation of treatment with an IR preparation, before switching to the modified-release formulation.

Diuretics, loop

CLINICAL PHARMACOLOGY

Common indications	❶ For relief of breathlessness in **acute pulmonary oedema** in conjunction with <u>oxygen</u> and <u>nitrates</u>. ❷ For symptomatic treatment of fluid overload in **chronic heart failure.** ❸ For symptomatic treatment of fluid overload in **other oedematous states,** e.g. due to renal disease or liver failure, where they may be given in combination with other diuretics.
Mechanisms of action	As their name suggests, loop diuretics act principally on the ascending limb of the **loop of Henle,** where they **inhibit the Na⁺/K⁺/2Cl⁻ co-transporter.** This protein is responsible for transporting sodium, potassium and chloride ions from the tubular lumen into the epithelial cell. Water then follows by osmosis. Inhibiting this process has a potent diuretic effect. In addition, loop diuretics have a direct effect on blood vessels, causing **dilatation of capacitance veins.** In acute heart failure, this reduces preload and improves contractile function of the 'overstretched' heart muscle. Indeed, this is probably the main benefit of loop diuretics in acute heart failure, as illustrated by the fact that the clinical response is usually evident before a diuresis is established.
Important adverse effects	Water losses due to diuresis can lead to **dehydration** and **hypotension.** Inhibiting the Na⁺/K⁺/2Cl⁻ co-transporter increases urinary losses of sodium, potassium and chloride ions. Indirectly, this also increases excretion of magnesium, calcium and hydrogen ions. You can therefore associate loop diuretics with almost any **low electrolyte state** (i.e. hyponatraemia, hypokalaemia, hypochloraemia, hypocalcaemia, hypomagnesaemia and metabolic alkalosis). A similar Na⁺/K⁺/2Cl⁻ co-transporter is responsible for regulating endolymph composition in the inner ear. At high doses, loop diuretics can affect this too, leading to **hearing loss** and **tinnitus.**
Warnings	Loop diuretics are contraindicated in patients with severe ✖**hypovolemia** or ✖**dehydration**. They should be used with caution in patients at risk of ▲**hepatic encephalopathy** (where hypokalaemia can cause or worsen coma) and those with severe ▲**hypokalaemia** and/or ▲**hyponatraemia.** Taken chronically, loop diuretics inhibit uric acid excretion and this can worsen ▲**gout.**
Important interactions	Loop diuretics have the potential to affect **drugs that are excreted by the kidneys.** For example, ▲lithium levels are increased due to reduced excretion. The risk of ▲digoxin toxicity may also be increased, due to the effects of diuretic-associated hypokalaemia. Loop diuretics can increase the ototoxicity and nephrotoxicity of ▲<u>aminoglycosides</u>.

PRACTICAL PRESCRIBING

Prescription	Loop diuretics are available in oral and IV preparations. In the management of acute pulmonary oedema, you usually prescribe the initial dose of the loop diuretic intravenously, due to its more rapid and reliable effect. A typical choice is furosemide 40 mg IV, prescribed in the once-only section. Then, depending on your patient's response (see Monitoring), you may need to prescribe additional IV bolus doses, regular oral maintenance doses or, in resistant cases, an IV infusion.
Administration	Intravenous doses of furosemide should be administered slowly, at a rate no greater than 4 mg/min. Oral maintenance doses should be taken in the morning (with a second dose in the early afternoon in the case of twice daily administration) to avoid causing nocturia.
Communication	Explain to your patient that their body is overloaded with water. You are therefore offering a treatment to increase urine flow, which will hopefully improve this. The medicine will inevitably cause them to need to **pass water more often.** Provided they do not take doses late in the day it should not affect them at night.
Monitoring	For **efficacy** in the acute management of pulmonary oedema, evidence for a good response will include improvements in the patient's symptoms, tachycardia, hypertension and oxygen requirement. Increased urine output typically occurs later and indicates onset of the diuretic effect. In longer-term therapy, you should monitor your patient's symptoms, signs and body weight (aiming for losses of no more than 1 kg/day). For **safety,** periodic monitoring of serum sodium, potassium and renal function is also advisable, particularly in the first few weeks of therapy.
Cost	In tablet and injectable forms, furosemide and bumetanide are cheap. Oral solutions are considerably more expensive (about 20 times more in the case of furosemide; over 100 times for bumetanide).

Clinical tip—The proportion of furosemide absorbed from the gut (i.e. its *bioavailability*) is highly variable, both between and within individuals. It tends to be particularly low in the context of severe fluid overload, presumably due to gut wall oedema. This problem can be circumvented by administering furosemide IV, but this will not always be possible or desirable. In such cases, bumetanide may be a better choice, as its bioavailability is more predictable. Bumetanide 1 mg is equivalent to about 40 mg of furosemide.

Diuretics, potassium-sparing

CLINICAL PHARMACOLOGY

Common indications	❶ As part of combination therapy, for the treatment of **hypokalaemia** arising from <u>loop-</u> or <u>thiazide-diuretic</u> therapy. <u>Aldosterone antagonists</u> (e.g. spironolactone) also have a potassium-sparing effect, and may be used as an alternative.
Mechanisms of action	Potassium-sparing diuretics such as amiloride are relatively **weak diuretics alone.** However, in combination with another diuretic, they can **counteract potassium loss** and enhance diuresis. Amiloride acts on the **distal convoluted tubules** in the kidney. It inhibits the reabsorption of sodium (and therefore water) by epithelial sodium channels (ENaC), leading to sodium and water excretion, and retention of potassium. This counteracts the potassium losses associated with loop- or thiazide-diuretic therapy. Amiloride is available as a medicine in its own right, but tends more often to be used as part of a combination tablet with furosemide (a <u>loop diuretic</u>) as co-amilofruse, or with hydrochlorothiazide (a <u>thiazide diuretic</u>) as co-amilozide. The ratio of the two drugs in the combination tablets is designed to have a neutral effect on potassium balance, although in practice this may not always be the case.
Important adverse effects	Side effects are uncommon at low doses, but **gastrointestinal upset** may occur. When used in combination with other diuretics, dizziness, **hypotension** and **urinary symptoms** may be problematic. As combined preparations, **electrolyte disturbances** should cancel each other out, but the risk of hypokalaemia, hyperkalaemia and hyponatraemia should not be ignored.
Warnings	Avoid in ✖**severe renal impairment** and ✖**hyperkalaemia.** Combination therapy should not be started in the context of ▲**hypokalaemia,** as the effect on potassium may be unpredictable. As with all diuretics, they should be avoided in states of ▲**volume depletion.**
Important interactions	Do not use in combination with other ▲**potassium-elevating drugs,** including ✖<u>potassium supplements (oral or IV)</u> and ✖<u>aldosterone antagonists</u>, due to the risk of hyperkalaemia. As with other diuretics, renal clearance of drugs including ▲<u>digoxin</u> and ▲lithium may be altered, requiring dose adjustment.

amiloride (as co-amilofruse, co-amilozide)

PRACTICAL PRESCRIBING

Prescription	The most commonly used product is co-amilofruse, a tablet containing furosemide and amiloride in a ratio of 1:8. It is important to **state the 'strength' of the tablet** (i.e. their drug content) on the prescription. This is specified as, for example, 'co-amilofruse 2.5/20', meaning that the tablet contains 2.5 mg of amiloride and 20 mg of furosemide. You then **state the dose as the number of tablets** to be taken daily. The strength and dose are usually selected to match the dose of the existing loop or thiazide diuretic. So, for example, if you have a patient currently taking furosemide 40 mg daily (which is controlling their symptoms but causing hypokalaemia), you might replace this with co-amilofruse 5/40, 1 tablet daily.
Administration	It is best to take diuretic tablets in the morning, to minimise nocturia.
Communication	Explain that their potassium level is low because of the water tablet they are already taking. You are now offering to change to a different water tablet, which contains another medicine that will hopefully prevent the loss of potassium. Warn them of common side effects, such as increased **urinary frequency** and **gastrointestinal upset.** Ensure they understand the **importance of blood test monitoring,** to check that their potassium level returns to normal.
Monitoring	The best form of monitoring for efficacy is the patient's **symptoms** of fluid overload (in the case of co-amilofruse) or their blood pressure (for co-amilozide). You should monitor their serum **potassium** concentration to ensure this returns to normal. The intensity of biochemical monitoring will depend on the severity of the hypokalaemia.
Cost	Co-amilofruse and co-amilozide are available in non-proprietary forms and are relatively inexpensive. However, the higher strength co-amilofruse tablets (co-amilofruse 10/80) are significantly more expensive than the lower strength forms (2.5/20 and 5/40).

Clinical tip—Aldosterone stimulates sodium (and water) absorption in the late distal tubule by activating epithelial sodium channels (ENaC). Sodium absorption through ENaC is inhibited directly by amiloride and indirectly by spironolactone, which blocks aldosterone receptors. Amiloride may therefore be a useful alternative to spironolactone, for example in the treatment of hypertension due to hyperaldosteronism (Conn's syndrome) or added to loop or thiazide diuretics, particularly where adverse effects of spironolactone (such as gynaecomastia) are unacceptable.

Diuretics, thiazide and thiazide-like

CLINICAL PHARMACOLOGY

Common indications	❶ Thiazides are an **alternative first-line treatment for hypertension** where a calcium channel blocker would otherwise be used, but is either unsuitable (e.g. due to oedema) or there are features of heart failure. ❷ Thiazides are also an **add-on treatment for hypertension** in patients whose blood pressure is not adequately controlled by a calcium channel blocker plus an ACE inhibitor or angiotensin receptor blocker (ARB).
Mechanisms of action	Thiazide diuretics (e.g. bendroflumethiazide) and thiazide-like diuretics (e.g. indapamide, chlortalidone) differ chemically but have similar effects and uses; we refer to them collectively as 'thiazides.' **Thiazides inhibit the Na^+/Cl^- co-transporter in the distal convoluted tubule of the nephron.** This prevents reabsorption of sodium and its osmotically associated water. The resulting diuresis causes an initial fall in extracellular fluid volume. Over time, compensatory changes (e.g. activation of the renin–angiotensin system) tend to reverse this, at least in part. The long-term antihypertensive effect is probably mediated by **vasodilatation,** the mechanism of which is incompletely understood.
Important adverse effects	Preventing sodium ion reabsorption from the nephron can cause **hyponatraemia,** although this is not usually problematic. The increased delivery of sodium to the distal tubule, where it can be exchanged for potassium, increases urinary potassium losses and may therefore cause **hypokalaemia.** This, in turn, may cause **cardiac arrhythmias.** Thiazides may increase plasma concentrations of glucose (which may unmask type 2 diabetes), LDL-cholesterol and triglycerides. However, their net effect on cardiovascular risk is protective. They may cause **impotence** in men.
Warnings	Thiazides should be avoided in patients with ✖**hypokalaemia** and ▲**hyponatraemia.** As they reduce uric acid excretion, they may precipitate acute attacks in patients with ▲**gout.**
Important interactions	The effectiveness of thiazides may be reduced by non-steroidal anti-inflammatory drugs (although low-dose aspirin is not a concern). The combination of thiazides with other drugs that lower the serum potassium concentration (e.g. ▲loop diuretics) is best avoided. If combination is essential, it should prompt intensive electrolyte monitoring.

bendroflumethiazide, indapamide, chlortalidone

PRACTICAL PRESCRIBING

Prescription	Thiazides are taken orally as part of the patient's regular medication. Indapamide (e.g. 2.5 mg daily) and chlortalidone (12.5–25 mg daily) are recommended for hypertension. Historically in UK practice, bendroflumethiazide 2.5 mg daily has been widely used, but this is less desirable as there are no supporting clinical trials to confirm its benefit. There is little to be gained from higher dose treatment, as this tends just to increase side effects without significantly improving the antihypertensive effect.
Administration	It is generally best to take the tablet in the morning, so that the diuretic effect is maximal during the day rather than at night and does not therefore interfere with sleep.
Communication	Explain to your patient that you are offering treatment with a 'water tablet' for their high blood pressure. If they have leg swelling, it may also help with this. Enquire whether they have any difficulty getting to the toilet in time (either because of mobility issues or sensations of urgency), since the water tablet is likely to make them pass water more often. Advise patients that anti-inflammatory drugs like ibuprofen, which can be bought without prescription, may interact with water tablets and interfere with the way they work. At review, ask men directly about the possible side effect of impotence, as this may not be volunteered without prompting.
Monitoring	The best measure of efficacy is the patient's blood pressure and, if applicable, the severity of their oedema. Measure the patient's serum electrolyte concentrations before starting the drug, at 2–4 weeks into therapy, and after any change in therapy that might alter electrolyte balance.
Cost	Indapamide, chlortalidone and bendroflumethiazide are available in non-proprietary forms and are inexpensive. Indapamide is also available in branded modified-release forms. These are more expensive but there is no convincing evidence that they are clinically superior.

Clinical tip—One of the main adverse effects of thiazides is *hypokalaemia,* while one of the main adverse effects of ACE inhibitors and ARBs is *hyperkalaemia.* Moreover, these drug classes have a synergistic blood pressure lowering effect: thiazides tend to activate the renin–angiotensin system, while ACE inhibitors/ARBs block it. Consequently, the combination of a thiazide and an ACE inhibitor/ARB is very useful in practice, both to improve blood pressure control and to maintain neutral potassium balance.

Dopaminergic drugs for Parkinson's disease

CLINICAL PHARMACOLOGY

Common indications	❶ Dopaminergic drugs are used in **early Parkinson's disease,** when dopamine agonists (e.g. ropinirole, pramipexol) may be preferred over levodopa. ❷ In **later Parkinson's disease,** levodopa is an integral part of management, while dopamine agonists are an option for add-on therapy. ❸ Levodopa and dopamine agonists may be options for **secondary parkinsonism** (parkinsonian symptoms due to a cause other than idiopathic Parkinson's disease), but addressing the underlying cause (e.g. discontinuation of an offending drug) generally takes precedence.
Mechanisms of action	In Parkinson's disease, there is a **deficiency of dopamine in the nigrostriatal pathway** that links the substantia nigra in the midbrain to the corpus striatum in the basal ganglia. Via direct and indirect circuits, this causes the basal ganglia to exert greater inhibitory effects on the thalamus which, in turn, reduces excitatory input to the motor cortex. This generates the features of Parkinson's disease, such as bradykinesia and rigidity. Treatment seeks to increase dopaminergic stimulation to the striatum. It is not possible to give dopamine itself because it does not cross the blood–brain barrier. By contrast, levodopa (L-dopa) is a **precursor of dopamine** that can enter the brain via a membrane transporter. Ropinirole and pramipexol are relatively selective **agonists for the D_2 receptor,** which predominates in the striatum.
Important adverse effects	All dopaminergic drugs can cause **nausea, drowsiness, confusion, hallucinations** and **hypotension.** A major problem with levodopa is the **wearing-off effect,** where the patient's symptoms worsen towards the end of the dosage interval. This seems to get worse as duration of therapy increases. It can be partially overcome by increasing the dose and/or frequency, but this can generate the opposite effect: excessive and involuntary movements **(dyskinesias)** at the beginning of the dosage interval. When these occur together, this is called the **on–off effect.**
Warnings	Dopaminergic drugs should be used cautiously in the ▲**elderly** and those with ▲**existing cognitive or psychiatric disease,** due to the risk of causing confusion and hallucinations. They should also be used cautiously in those with ▲**cardiovascular disease,** because of the risk of hypotension.
Important interactions	Levodopa is always given with a peripheral dopa-decarboxylase inhibitor (e.g. carbidopa) to reduce its conversion to dopamine outside the brain. This desirable interaction reduces nausea and lowers the dose needed for therapeutic effect. Dopaminergic agents should not usually be combined with ▲antipsychotics (particularly first-generation) or ▲metoclopramide because their effects on dopamine receptors are contradictory.

levodopa (as co-careldopa, co-beneldopa), ropinirole, pramipexol

PRACTICAL PRESCRIBING

Prescription	Starting or altering pharmacological therapy in **Parkinson's disease** should be done only under specialist advice. Many specialists prefer dopamine agonists in early disease then add levodopa when symptoms become disabling. The aim of this is to defer development of on–off effects until as late as possible. Levodopa is only available in combined preparations with peripheral dopa-decarboxylase inhibitors: with benserazide (co-beneldopa) or carbidopa (co-careldopa).
Administration	It is very important with levodopa that doses are taken at times that produce the best symptom control for the patient. This is especially important if the patient is admitted to hospital (see Clinical tip).
Communication	Close communication is essential between the patient and specialists in Parkinson's disease. Often a clinical nurse specialist will form the vital link in this partnership. You should engage with the specialist team to support this.
Monitoring	The best form of monitoring for clinical efficacy and side effects is an assessment by a Parkinson's disease specialist. Blood pressure should be monitored in all patients receiving dopaminergic therapy, particularly those with existing cardiovascular disease.
Cost	The dopaminergic drugs mentioned here are available in non-proprietary forms. Although not inexpensive, these are less expensive than their brand name equivalents. However, there may be good reasons to use a branded product in some cases (e.g. when the on–off effect is prominent, switching to a modified-release form may mitigate this). You should not alter the brand of a patient's anti-parkinsonism medicine without discussion with a specialist.

Clinical tip—As a foundation doctor you are unlikely to play a major role in active prescribing decisions regarding anti-parkinsonian therapy. However, you may be integral in *ensuring that the patient's therapy is maintained* if they are admitted to hospital. Adhering to the correct timing of doses is essential: ask the patient exactly what time they take each dose and prescribe accordingly. Discuss the importance of this with nursing staff and, where appropriate, consider implementing a self-medication approach. You should also know that dopaminergic therapy should never be stopped abruptly. As well as causing an inevitable deterioration in symptom control, there is a risk that this may precipitate neuroleptic malignant syndrome. In patients who become unable to take tablets, a transdermal dopamine-agonist preparation may be useful.

Emollients

CLINICAL PHARMACOLOGY

Common indications	❶ As a topical treatment for all **dry** or **scaling skin disorders.** Specifically, they are used alone or in combination with <u>topical corticosteroids</u> in the treatment of **eczema.** They can reduce skin dryness and cracking in **psoriasis,** where, depending on severity, they are used alone or in combination with other therapies.
Mechanisms of action	Emollients help to **replace water** content in dry skin. They contain oils or paraffin-based products that help to soften the skin and can **reduce water loss** by protecting against evaporation from the skin surface. Many preparations can be used as a soap substitute (as soap is drying to the skin) and there are also specific bath or shower emollient preparations available.
Important adverse effects	Emollients have few adverse effects. The main tolerability issue is that they cause **greasiness** of the skin, but this is integral to their therapeutic effect. Emollient ointments can **exacerbate acne vulgaris** and **folliculitis** by blocking pores and hair follicles.
Warnings	While these drugs are usually very safe to use, paraffin-based emollients are a significant **fire hazard** when the oil content is high (>50%).
Important interactions	There are no significant interactions with other medications. However, when using more than one topical product, applications should be spaced out. This ensures that small volumes of topical drugs (e.g. topical corticosteroids) are not prevented from reaching the affected skin by large quantities of emollient.

PRACTICAL PRESCRIBING

Prescription	Emollients are emulsions of oil and water formulated as semi-solid **creams** (50% oil, 50% water), semi-liquid **lotions** (less oil, more water) or **ointments** (80% oil, 20% water). The choice of preparation will depend on the amount of skin to cover (lotions and creams spread further) and the severity of the condition (ointments are more occlusive and potent and last longer), as well as patient preference. You should prescribe emollients to be applied at least two or three times a day in active disease as their effect is quite short lasting. **You should prescribe large volumes,** e.g. 500 g, to ensure a sufficient supply for frequent and widespread application. Treatment should continue after improvement of symptoms to prevent recurrence.
Administration	Apply emollients in the direction of hair growth to reduce the risk of folliculitis.
Communication	Explain that you are offering a therapy that should improve skin dryness, but that it may take several days or weeks of treatment for the full effect to be seen. Encourage patients to apply emollients as often as possible. Advise them to use emollients instead of soap for hand-washing as well as when washing in a bath or shower. Warn them that **emollients can make bathroom fittings slippery.** When treating **eczema,** advise the patient to apply emollient to the whole body, rather than just the affected skin, and to keep using emollients even when the disease is controlled, to stop it returning. If they are using other topical agents, advise them to apply these first and leave 5 minutes before applying an emollient.
Monitoring	When treating conditions like **eczema** or **psoriasis** you should review the patient to determine whether therapy has been effective. If emollients are ineffective, you may need to prescribe a second agent, such as a topical corticosteroid.
Cost	Non-proprietary emollients are cheap, around £2–£5 for 500 g. Proprietary preparations are often double this.

Clinical tip—Most people who find emollients ineffective are not applying them frequently enough. Sometimes this is because they find them greasy and unpleasant. In this case encourage them to try a cream or a lotion instead of an ointment and apply the treatment more often.

Fibrinolytic drugs

CLINICAL PHARMACOLOGY

Common indications	❶ In **acute ischaemic stroke,** *alteplase* increases the chance of living independently if it is given within 4.5 hours of the onset of the stroke. ❷ In **acute ST elevation myocardial infarction,** *alteplase* and *streptokinase* can reduce mortality when they are given within 12 hours of the onset of symptoms in combination with antiplatelet agents and anticoagulants. However, primary percutaneous coronary intervention (where available) has largely superseded fibrinolytics in this context. ❸ For **massive pulmonary embolism with haemodynamic instability** fibrinolytic drugs reduce clot size and pulmonary artery pressures, but there is no clear evidence that they improve mortality.
Mechanisms of action	Fibrinolytic drugs, also known as thrombolytic drugs, catalyse the conversion of plasminogen to plasmin, which acts to **dissolve fibrinous clots** and **re-canalise occluded vessels.** This allows reperfusion of affected tissue, preventing or limiting tissue infarction and cell death and improving patient outcomes.
Important adverse effects	Common adverse effects include **nausea** and **vomiting, bruising** around the injection site and **hypotension.** Adverse effects that require treatment to be stopped include **serious bleeding, allergic reaction, cardiogenic shock** and **cardiac arrest.** Serious bleeding may require treatment with coagulation factors and antifibrinolytic drugs, e.g. tranexamic acid, but this is usually avoidable as fibrinolytic agents have a very short half-life. Reperfusion of infarcted brain or heart tissue can lead to **cerebral oedema** and **arrhythmias,** respectively.
Warnings	There are many contraindications to thrombolysis, which are mostly factors that predispose to ✖**bleeding** including: recent haemorrhage; recent trauma or surgery; bleeding disorders; severe hypertension; and peptic ulcers. In acute stroke, ✖**intracranial haemorrhage** must be excluded with a CT scan before treatment. ✖**Previous streptokinase treatment** is a contraindication to repeat dosing (although other fibrinolytics can be used), as development of anti-streptokinase antibodies can block its effect.
Important interactions	The risk of haemorrhage is increased in patients taking anticoagulants, and antiplatelet agents. <u>ACE inhibitors</u> appear to increase the risk of anaphylactoid reactions.

PRACTICAL PRESCRIBING

Prescription	Fibrinolytic drugs should only be prescribed by those experienced in their use. The dose varies depending on the indication, timing from the onset of symptoms and the patient's weight. They are only available as injectable preparations. A bolus dose is usually given first, followed by an IV infusion.
Administration	Fibrinolytic drugs should be administered in a high dependency area such as the emergency department, hyperacute stroke unit or coronary care unit, by staff experienced in their use. Alteplase comes as a powder, which is reconstituted with water for injection then either given directly as an IV bolus injection or diluted further in 0.9% sodium chloride and given as an IV infusion.
Communication	The decision to 'thrombolyse' (prescribe fibrinolytic therapy) should be made by a senior clinician and the risks and benefits discussed with the patient and next of kin. For example, in acute stroke, explain that part of the brain is being starved of blood and oxygen due to a blocked artery, which will cause long-term damage. Giving a 'clot-busting' drug can prevent damage to the brain by dissolving the blood clot and restoring blood flow. However, it only works when given soon after the onset of the stroke. With or without treatment people may show some improvement, but symptoms may also get worse and one in three strokes are fatal. Although the chance of death is increased initially after receiving a clot-busting drug (due to bleeding), after the first week the chances of living independently are increased. For licensed indications, written consent is not essential but verbal consent should be obtained. If neurological impairment prevents consent, treatment can still be given if judged to be in the patient's best interests.
Monitoring	Patients should be monitored in a high dependency area, with vital signs checked every 15 minutes for the first 2 hours. This should include observation for signs of bleeding, anaphylaxis and, in the case of acute stroke, neurological deterioration.
Cost	Fibrinolytic agents are currently only available as branded products. Treatment with alteplase costs around £300–£600 and with streptokinase costs around £80.

Clinical tip—In patients with acute ischaemic stroke, likely benefits of thrombolysis diminish rapidly with time. Compared to untreated patients, the chance of being alive and independent at 6 months is increased by 10% for patients who receive thrombolysis within 3 hours of symptom onset, but by 2% if thrombolysis is performed between 3 and 6 hours. Campaigns that encourage patients to present early, rapid triage and CT scanning and good organisation of thrombolysis services are essential for treatment to be effective.

Gabapentin and pregabalin

CLINICAL PHARMACOLOGY

Common indications	❶ Both drugs are used for **focal epilepsies** (with or without secondary generalisation), usually as an add-on treatment when other antiepileptic drugs (e.g. <u>carbamazepine</u>) provide inadequate control. ❷ Both drugs are used for **neuropathic pain;** pregabalin in particular is recommended as a second-line option in painful diabetic neuropathy (after duloxetine) and as a first-line option in other painful neuropathies. ❸ Gabapentin is used in **migraine prophylaxis.** ❹ Pregabalin is used in **generalised anxiety disorder.**
Mechanisms of action	From a structural point of view, gabapentin is closely related to γ-aminobutyric acid (GABA), the major inhibitory neurotransmitter in the brain. However, its mechanism of action, although not completely understood, appears largely unrelated to GABA. It binds with **voltage-sensitive calcium (Ca^{2+}) channels,** where it presumably prevents inflow of Ca^{2+} and, in so doing, inhibits neurotransmitter release. This interferes with synaptic transmission and reduces neuronal excitability. Pregabalin is a structural analogue of gabapentin that probably has a similar mechanism of action.
Important adverse effects	Gabapentin and pregabalin are generally better tolerated than other antiepileptic drugs. Their main side effects are **drowsiness, dizziness** and **ataxia,** which usually improve over the first few weeks of treatment.
Warnings	Both drugs depend on the kidneys for their elimination, so their doses should be reduced in ▲**renal impairment.**
Important interactions	The sedative effects of gabapentin and pregabalin may be enhanced when combined with other ▲**sedating drugs** (e.g. <u>benzodiazepines</u>). Other than this, gabapentin and pregabalin are notable in having relatively few drug interactions – in stark contrast to most other antiepileptic drugs. This makes them particularly useful where combination regimens are considered necessary.

gabapentin, pregabalin

PRACTICAL PRESCRIBING

Prescription	Gabapentin and pregabalin are taken orally. To improve tolerability, they should be started at a low dose. The dose is then increased over subsequent days and weeks to reach a dose that strikes the optimal balance between benefits and side effects. Appropriate escalating-dose regimens are listed in the BNF.
Administration	There are no special considerations with regard to the oral administration of gabapentin and pregabalin.
Communication	Explain that you are offering a medicine which you anticipate will reduce the severity of their symptoms (e.g. the frequency of their fits). Explain that the medicine commonly causes some drowsiness or dizziness. For this reason, you will prescribe a low dose initially, then increase this gradually (make sure they are clear on the dosing instructions). Explain that these side effects should improve over the first few weeks. They should avoid driving or operating machines until they are confident that the symptoms have settled.
Monitoring	The best guide to clinical effectiveness is to enquire about symptoms (e.g. seizure frequency) and side effects. There is no need to monitor serum/plasma concentrations of gabapentin or pregabalin.
Cost	Gabapentin is available in both branded and non-proprietary forms. In spite of containing the same chemical, the brand name product is significantly more expensive; there is no reason to prefer it. At the time of writing, pregabalin is only available as an expensive branded product.

Clinical tip—Gabapentin may cause false-positive results for detection of protein on urine dipstick testing. In this case, a sample should be sent to the laboratory for quantitative analysis (e.g. a spot sample for protein:creatinine ratio), which is not affected by gabapentin.

H₂-receptor antagonists

CLINICAL PHARMACOLOGY

Common indications	**❶ Peptic ulcer disease:** for treatment and prevention of gastric and duodenal ulcers and NSAID-associated ulcers, although proton pump inhibitors (PPIs) are more effective and therefore usually preferred. **❷ Gastro-oesophageal reflux disease (GORD)** and **dyspepsia:** for relief of symptoms. PPIs are the main alternative, and are preferred in more severe cases.
Mechanisms of action	Histamine H₂-receptor antagonists ('H₂-blockers') **reduce gastric acid secretion.** Acid is normally produced by the proton pump of the gastric parietal cell, which secretes H⁺ into the stomach lumen in exchange for drawing K⁺ into the cell. The proton pump is regulated, among other things, by histamine. Histamine is released by local paracrine cells and binds to H₂-receptors on the gastric parietal cell. Via a second-messenger system, this activates the proton pump. Blocking H₂-receptors therefore reduces acid secretion. However, as the proton pump can also be stimulated by other pathways, H₂-blockers cannot completely suppress gastric acid production. In this respect they differ from PPIs, which tend to have a more complete suppressive effect.
Important adverse effects	H₂-blockers are generally well tolerated with **few side effects.** Most common among these are bowel disturbance (diarrhoea or, less often, constipation), headache and dizziness.
Warnings	H₂-blockers are excreted by the kidneys, so their dose should be reduced in patients with renal impairment. Like PPIs, they can **disguise the symptoms of gastric cancer,** so it is important not just to treat symptoms without considering and, if appropriate, investigating their cause.
Important interactions	Ranitidine has **no major drug interactions.**

PRACTICAL PRESCRIBING

Prescription	Ranitidine can be purchased over the counter, but only for short-term use. You will need to write a prescription if you intend for the patient to take it for more than 2 weeks. The dose varies according to the indication, but 150 mg twice daily is typical. Likewise, the duration of therapy varies according to the indication.
Administration	Oral preparations can be taken before, with or after food.
Communication	Explain that you are offering treatment to reduce stomach acid. This will hopefully improve their symptoms and, if applicable, allow their ulcer to heal. It is reasonable to say that side effects are pretty uncommon with this medicine. Ensure that both you and the patient are clear on the intended duration of therapy and the need to report any 'alarm' symptoms (e.g. weight loss, swallowing difficulty), should they arise.
Monitoring	For treatment of peptic ulcer disease, repeat endoscopy may be necessary in some cases to confirm healing. For symptomatic treatment of dyspepsia and GORD, the patient's symptoms are the best guide to the effect of therapy.
Cost	Standard ranitidine tablets are inexpensive; effervescent tablets and oral solution are about ten times more expensive.

Clinical tip—H_2-blockers have been superseded by PPIs for most indications, due to their more complete acid suppressing effect. One advantage that H_2-blockers retain, however, is a more rapid onset of effect. This probably makes them a better choice for suppressing gastric acid production pre-operatively. In a patient with significant GORD due to undergo general anaesthesia, there is a risk that gastric acid may reflux and then be aspirated, causing pneumonitis. The anaesthetist may prescribe a dose of ranitidine in an attempt to mitigate this. You may score brownie points if you identify such patients and prescribe ranitidine yourself. You are looking for patients with active reflux symptoms – the sensation of acid coming up the gullet – who are due to undergo a procedure involving sedation or general anaesthesia. Offer ranitidine 300 mg orally, to be taken with a sip of water at least 2 hours before the start of the surgical list.

Heparins and fondaparinux

CLINICAL PHARMACOLOGY

Common indications	❶ **Venous thromboembolism (VTE):** low molecular weight heparin (LMWH) is the first choice agent for pharmacological VTE prophylaxis in hospital inpatients, and for initial treatment of **deep vein thrombosis** (DVT) and **pulmonary embolism** (PE). ❷ **Acute coronary syndrome (ACS):** LMWH or fondaparinux are part of first-line therapy to improve revascularisation and prevent intracoronary thrombus progression.
Mechanisms of action	**Thrombin** and **factor Xa** are key components of the **final common coagulation pathway** that leads to formation of a fibrin clot. By inhibiting their function, heparins and fondaparinux prevent the formation and propagation of blood clots. Unfractionated heparin (UFH) activates antithrombin that, in turn, **inactivates clotting factor Xa and thrombin. Low molecular weight heparins** such as dalteparin and enoxaparin have a similar mechanism of action but **preferentially inhibit factor Xa.** Low molecular weight heparins have a more predictable effect and, unlike UFH, do not usually require laboratory monitoring. Consequently, LMWHs are now preferred in most indications. **Fondaparinux** is a synthetic compound that is similar to heparin. It **inhibits factor Xa only.** It appears to have similar efficacy to LMWH and has become the anticoagulant of choice in the treatment of ACS in many hospitals in the UK.
Important adverse effects	The main adverse effect of heparins and fondaparinux is **bleeding.** This risk may be lower with fondaparinux than with LMWH or UFH. As with many injectables, these drugs may cause **injection site reactions.** Rarely, heparins may cause a dangerous syndrome characterised by low platelet count and thrombosis **(heparin-induced thrombocytopenia).** This immune reaction is less likely with LMWH and fondaparinux than UFH.
Warnings	Anticoagulants should be used with caution in patients at increased risk of bleeding, including those with ▲**clotting disorders,** ▲**severe uncontrolled hypertension,** or ▲**recent surgery or trauma.** Heparins should be avoided around the time of ▲**invasive procedures,** particularly lumbar puncture and spinal anaesthesia. In patients with ▲**renal impairment,** LMWH and fondaparinux may accumulate and should be used at a lower dose, or unfractionated heparin used instead.
Important interactions	Combining antithrombotic drugs increases the risk of bleeding. This should usually be avoided unless there is a special reason for combined therapy, such as in the use of LMWH while initiating <u>warfarin</u>, or the use of antiplatelet drugs (e.g. <u>aspirin</u>, <u>clopidogrel</u>) with fondaparinux/LMWH in ACS. In major bleeding associated with heparin therapy, protamine can be given to reverse anticoagulation. This is effective for UFH but much less so for LMWH. It is ineffective against fondaparinux.

enoxaparin, dalteparin, fondaparinux, unfractionated heparin

PRACTICAL PRESCRIBING

Prescription	LMWH and fondaparinux are prescribed for regular administration. Some hospitals have a dedicated prescription chart for anticoagulants. They are given by SC injection. The dose is dependent on indication and the patient's weight. For **prophylaxis of VTE** in medical inpatients, common choices are enoxaparin 40 mg SC daily or dalteparin 5000 units SC daily. Higher doses are used in **treatment of VTE and ACS.** UFH is sometimes given by IV infusion, and is therefore prescribed in the infusion section of the chart. This is complicated and you should refer to a local protocol.
Administration	SC injections of these drugs should be given into the subcutaneous tissue of the abdominal wall. The arm should not be used because this can cause uncomfortable and disabling bruising.
Communication	In the context of VTE prophylaxis, explain that you are offering a daily injection that will reduce the risk of blood clots. In longer-term therapy (e.g. for the treatment of VTE in cancer, when LMWH may be preferred over warfarin), discuss the risks and benefits of anticoagulation. Advise patients to avoid activities that may increase their risk of bleeding, such as contact sports, and to inform healthcare professionals they come into contact with that they are taking anticoagulants. If appropriate, train patients how to self-administer SC injections.
Monitoring	The activated partial thromboplastin ratio (APTR) indicates the anticoagulant effect of UFH and is measured frequently (e.g. every 6 hours initially) during an infusion of UFH. The infusion rate should be altered to achieve the target APTR (usually 1.5–2.5). The **anticoagulant effects of LMWH and fondaparinux rarely require monitoring.** If required (e.g. in pregnancy), LMWH can be monitored by anti-Xa activity. The full blood count and renal profile should be checked in all cases. In prolonged therapy (>4 days), **platelet count should be monitored.** If thrombocytopenia occurs, the drug must be stopped and specialist advice sought immediately.
Cost	UFH is relatively inexpensive. LMWH is more expensive and fondaparinux is the most expensive. However, health economic assessments suggest they are cost effective when used appropriately.

Clinical tip—Following a new diagnosis of VTE, patients will often be treated initially with LMWH *and* warfarin. This is because warfarin inhibits the natural anticoagulant activity of proteins C and S, and it does this before inhibiting the other clotting factors. Using LMWH provides anticoagulant 'cover' during this initial pro-coagulant period. LMWH is stopped when the patient's INR is in therapeutic range.

Insulin

CLINICAL PHARMACOLOGY

Common indications	❶ For insulin replacement in people with **type 1 diabetes mellitus** and control of blood glucose in people with **type 2 diabetes mellitus** where oral hypoglycaemic treatment is inadequate or poorly tolerated. ❷ Given intravenously, in the treatment of **diabetic emergencies** such as diabetic ketoacidosis and hyperglycaemic hyperosmolar syndrome, and for **perioperative glycaemic control** in *selected* diabetic patients. ❸ Alongside <u>glucose</u> to treat **hyperkalaemia**, while other measures (such as treatment of the underlying cause) are initiated.
Mechanisms of action	In **diabetes mellitus,** exogenous insulin **functions similarly to endogenous insulin.** It stimulates glucose uptake from the circulation into tissues, including skeletal muscle and fat, and increases use of glucose as an energy source. Insulin stimulates glycogen, lipid and protein synthesis and inhibits gluconeogenesis and ketogenesis. For the treatment of **hyperkalaemia, insulin drives K⁺ into cells,** reducing serum K⁺ concentrations. However, once insulin treatment is stopped, K⁺ leaks back out of the cells into the circulation, so this is a short-term measure while other treatment is commenced.
	The wide choice of insulin preparations for treatment of diabetes mellitus can be classified as: **rapid acting** (immediate onset, short duration): insulin aspart, e.g. Novorapid®; **short acting** (early onset, short duration): soluble insulin, e.g. Actrapid®; **intermediate acting** (intermediate onset and duration): isophane (NPH) insulin, e.g. Humulin I®; and **long acting** (flat profile with regular administration): insulin glargine (Lantus®), insulin detemir (Levemir®). **Biphasic insulin** preparations contain a mixture of rapid- and intermediate-acting insulins, e.g. Novomix® 30 (insulin aspart/insulin aspart protamine).
	Where IV insulin is required (hyperkalaemia, diabetic emergencies, peri-operative glucose control), soluble insulin (Actrapid®) is usually used.
Important adverse effects	The main adverse effect of insulin is **hypoglycaemia,** which can be severe enough to lead to coma and death. When administered by repeated subcutaneous (SC) injection at the same site, insulin can cause fat overgrowth (lipohypertrophy), which may be unsightly or uncomfortable.
Warnings	In patients with ▲**renal impairment,** insulin clearance is reduced, so there is an increased risk of hypoglycaemia.
Important interactions	Although often necessary, combining insulin with other hypoglycaemic agents increases the risk of hypoglycaemia. Concurrent therapy with <u>systemic corticosteroids</u> increases insulin requirements.

insulin aspart, insulin glargine, biphasic insulin, soluble insulin

PRACTICAL PRESCRIBING

Prescription	In **diabetes mellitus,** patients may self-administer regular insulin by SC injection. The goal of treatment is to attain good blood glucose control without problematic hypoglycaemia. Insulin treatment is prescribed in units. Normal daily requirement is ~30–50 units, although this varies considerably between individuals, depending on weight, diet and activity. Treatment usually includes once or twice daily long-acting insulin to meet basal requirements, with intermittent rapid or short-acting insulin injected with meals to control post-prandial glucose. *Example regimens*: insulin glargine once daily and insulin aspart with meals and snacks; or Novomix® 30 twice daily. In **diabetic emergencies** and **peri-operative glycaemic control,** 50 units of Actrapid® are diluted in 50 mL of 0.9% sodium chloride to a concentration of 1 unit/mL. Insulin is infused with IV fluids and <u>potassium</u> at a rate determined by the blood glucose concentration (consult a local hospital protocol). In **hyperkalaemia,** Actrapid® 10 units added to 20% <u>glucose</u> 100 mL and infused over 15 minutes is reasonable. It is essential that glucose is given with insulin for this indication to avoid hypoglycaemia.
Administration	SC insulin is often administered using 'pens' containing insulin in solution (100 units/mL). These allow a patient to 'dial up' the number of units required and administer insulin discreetly, e.g. through clothes.
Communication	When starting a patient with diabetes mellitus on insulin, explain that insulin will help to control blood sugar levels and prevent complications. Advise them that **lifestyle measures,** including a calorie-controlled diet and regular exercise, are needed as well as insulin to improve health. Warn them of the risk of **hypoglycaemia,** advising them of symptoms to watch out for (e.g. dizziness, agitation, nausea, sweating and confusion). Explain that, if hypoglycaemia develops, they should take something sugary (e.g. glucose tablets or a sugary drink) then something starchy, e.g. a sandwich.
Monitoring	Patients should measure capillary blood glucose regularly and adjust insulin dose based on results. **HbA$_{1c}$** (glycated haemoglobin) should be measured at least annually to assess long-term glycaemic control. Where insulin is given as a continuous IV infusion, serum K$^+$ should be measured at least every 4 hours to guide need for replacement.
Cost	Insulin costs the NHS >£300 million/year (the fourth biggest drug cost).

Clinical tip—Avoid using SC short-acting insulin (Actrapid®) to treat unexpected high blood glucose concentrations. Time to peak effect (2–3 hrs) is longer than commonly appreciated, and trying to correct hyperglycaemia quickly is often unnecessary and can be dangerous. Instead, try to understand *why* hyperglycaemia has occurred (e.g. infection) and make small alterations to the patient's regular insulin regimen.

Iron

CLINICAL PHARMACOLOGY

Common indications	❶ **Treatment of iron-deficiency anaemia.** ❷ **Prophylaxis of iron-deficiency anaemia** in patients with risk factors such as poor diet, malabsorption, menorrhagia, gastrectomy, haemodialysis and infants with low birth weight.
Mechanisms of action	The aim of iron therapy is to replenish iron stores. Iron is essential for erythropoiesis (the formation of new red blood cells). It is required for the synthesis of the haem component of haemoglobin, which gives red blood cells the ability to carry oxygen. Iron is best absorbed in its ferrous state (Fe^{2+}) in the duodenum and jejunum. Its absorption is increased by stomach acid and dietary acids such as ascorbic acid (vitamin C). Once absorbed into the blood stream, iron is bound by transferrin. Transferrin transports it either to be used in the bone marrow for erythropoiesis, or to be stored as ferritin in the liver, reticuloendothelial system, bone marrow, spleen and skeletal muscle.
Important adverse effects	The most common adverse effect of oral iron salts is **gastrointestinal upset,** including nausea, epigastric pain, constipation and diarrhoea. Patients may notice that their bowel motions turn black on treatment. Intravenous iron administration can cause injection site irritation and hypersensitivity reactions, including anaphylaxis.
Warnings	*Oral iron* therapy may exacerbate bowel symptoms in patients with ▲**intestinal disease,** including inflammatory bowel disease, diverticular disease and intestinal strictures. *Intravenous iron* should be used with caution in people with an ▲**atopic predisposition** due to the risk of anaphylactic reaction.
Important interactions	Oral iron salts can reduce the absorption of other drugs including <u>levothyroxine</u> and <u>bisphosphonates</u>. These medications should therefore be taken at least 2 hours before oral iron.

ferrous fumarate, ferrous sulfate

PRACTICAL PRESCRIBING

Prescription	Iron is available for oral or IV administration. Intravenous iron should be reserved for patients unable to tolerate sufficient oral iron to correct or prevent deficiency. It is also used for patients with end-stage renal disease, in whom it may be given with erythropoietin. Intravenous iron replacement does not lead to a more rapid increase in haemoglobin than oral iron.
	For **treatment of iron-deficiency anaemia,** you need to give 100–200 mg of elemental iron per day. Different oral iron preparations contain different amounts of elemental iron. For example, ferrous sulfate 200 mg contains 65 mg elemental iron. A prescription for ferrous sulfate 200 mg two to three times daily will therefore provide 130–195 mg elemental iron a day. Once the haemoglobin has returned to normal, continue the prescription for a further 3 months to replenish iron stores fully. For **prophylaxis of iron-deficiency anaemia,** ferrous sulfate 1–2 tablets daily should be sufficient. Gastrointestinal adverse effects may prevent patients from taking iron. Reducing the dose or switching to an alternative iron salt may improve tolerability.
Administration	Although oral iron salts are better absorbed on an empty stomach, they can be taken with food to reduce gastrointestinal side effects. Intravenous iron can be given as an injection over 10 minutes or as an infusion. Facilities for the management of anaphylaxis should be available.
Communication	Explain that treatment should top up their iron stores and improve symptoms of anaemia, but that it may take a few months before the full benefit is felt. Warn them that iron may turn their stools black. Advise them to come back if the iron upsets their stomach, as treatment can be changed to reduce side effects.
Monitoring	Monitor full blood count until the haemoglobin has returned to normal. You should expect to see the haemoglobin rise by around 20 g/L per month.
Cost	Ferrous sulfate and ferrous fumarate are both available in non-proprietary forms, are equally efficacious and are cheap. Brand name compound preparations with ascorbic acid and modified-release preparations have minimal additional clinical benefit for a considerable increase in cost.

Clinical tip—People with iron deficiency often require colonoscopy to investigate the cause of their anaemia. However, oral iron can turn stools black and sticky. This is problematic for visualising the bowel during lower gastrointestinal endoscopy as the sticky black stool coats the colon and obscures the endoscopist's view. Iron treatment should therefore be stopped for 7 days before the procedure.

Laxatives, bulk-forming

CLINICAL PHARMACOLOGY

Common indications	❶ **Constipation** and **faecal impaction,** particularly in patients who cannot increase their dietary fibre intake. ❷ **Mild chronic diarrhoea** associated with diverticular disease or irritable bowel syndrome.
Mechanisms of action	**Bulk-forming laxatives contain a hydrophilic substance,** such as a polysaccharide or cellulose, which is not absorbed or broken down in the gut. Like dietary fibre, **this attracts water into the stool** and increases its mass. Adequate fluid intake is therefore important to the action of bulk-forming laxatives. **Increased stool bulk stimulates peristalsis** and helps to relieve constipation. It can also help in chronic diarrhoea. This can be useful for some patients with diverticular disease, irritable bowel syndrome, or when managing stoma output.
Important adverse effects	These drugs are generally well tolerated, with mild **abdominal distension** and **flatulence** being the most common side effects. Rarely, but more seriously, they may cause **faecal impaction** and **gastrointestinal obstruction.**
Warnings	They should not be used in patients with subacute or established ✖**intestinal obstruction** or ▲**faecal impaction,** and in general should not be used in patients with ▲**ileus.**
Important interactions	There are no clinically significant adverse drug interactions with bulk-forming laxatives.

ispaghula husk, methylcellulose, sterculia

PRACTICAL PRESCRIBING

Prescription	Bulk-forming laxatives are prescribed on the regular section of the drug chart. You should prescribe them for administration around meal times. A common choice is ispaghula husk 1 sachet twice daily.
Administration	Bulk-forming laxatives may be provided in the form of granules or powder to be dissolved in water (ispaghula husk, sterculia) or tablets (methylcellulose). Importantly, they should be taken with plenty of water (at least 300 mL).
Communication	Explain that you are offering a laxative that works as a fibre supplement. This will hopefully make their stool easier to pass. Outline the common side effects. Tell them that the dose can be adjusted according to their symptoms, provided they do not exceed the maximum dose. Advise them to take the laxative with a meal and plenty of fluid. As bulk-forming laxatives absorb water, they should be stored in a dry place.
Monitoring	When treating inpatients, a stool chart is useful to monitor the effects of treatment. Outpatients can usually monitor and adjust their own treatment.
Cost	Bulk-forming laxatives are cheap: ispaghula husk costs less than 10p a sachet. Patients who need to pay for their prescription may save money if they buy it from a pharmacy.

Clinical tip—Do not routinely use bulk-forming laxatives for patients with new-onset constipation who have recently had abdominal surgery and may have surgical (paralytic) ileus, as they will be at increased risk of developing intestinal obstruction.

Laxatives, osmotic

CLINICAL PHARMACOLOGY

Common indications	❶ **Constipation** and **faecal impaction.** ❷ **Bowel preparation** prior to surgery or endoscopy. ❸ **Hepatic encephalopathy.**
Mechanisms of action	These medicines are based on **osmotically active substances** (sugars or alcohols) that are not digested or absorbed, and which therefore remain in the gut lumen. **They hold water in the stool,** maintaining its volume and **stimulating peristalsis.** Lactulose, in particular, also reduces ammonia absorption. It does this by increasing gut transit rate and acidifying the stool, which inhibits the proliferation of ammonia-producing bacteria. This is helpful in patients with liver failure, in whom ammonia plays a major role in the pathogenesis of hepatic encephalopathy.
Important adverse effects	**Flatulence, abdominal cramps** and **nausea** are common adverse effects, although they may decrease with time. As with other laxatives, **diarrhoea** is a possible complication. Phosphate enemas can cause **local irritation** and **electrolyte disturbances.**
Warnings	Osmotic laxatives are contraindicated in ✖**intestinal obstruction** as there is a risk of perforation. Phosphate enemas can cause significant fluid shifts so should be used with caution in ▲**heart failure,** ▲**ascites** and when ▲**electrolyte disturbances** are present.
Important interactions	There are no significant adverse drug interactions with osmotic laxatives, although the effects of ▲warfarin may be slightly increased.

lactulose, macrogol, phosphate enema

PRACTICAL PRESCRIBING

Prescription	Orally administered osmotic laxatives should generally be prescribed in the regular section of the drug chart. For example, when treating **constipation** or **faecal impaction** you might prescribe lactulose 15 mL twice daily, titrating this to response. Be aware that it may take a few days for an effect to be seen, as the drug needs to pass through the gastrointestinal tract to the colon. When using a phosphate enema to treat **faecal impaction,** prescribe it in the once-only or as-required section for rectal administration. The dose should not usually exceed one enema in 24 hours. For **bowel preparation,** you should refer to a local protocol for prescribing advice. When using lactulose to treat or prevent **hepatic encephalopathy,** you might start with 30–50 mL (doubled in constipation) three times daily, aiming for the patient to produce three soft/loose stools daily.
Administration	Osmotic laxatives may be taken with or without food. Oral solutions can be taken as they are or diluted in another liquid; powdered forms are dissolved in water. Enemas are administered with the patient lying on their side, as for a rectal examination. They should stay in this position for a few minutes or until they need to open their bowels.
Communication	Explain that you are offering treatment with a laxative that will hopefully make their stool softer and easier to pass. To work, it requires them to drink plenty of water: they should aim to have at least 6–8 glasses of liquid per day. Mention that side effects such as abdominal cramps and flatulence can occur, but these may get better over time. Advise that the dose should be adjusted to maintain comfort. If they are regularly passing more than two or three soft stools per day, the dose should definitely be reduced or the laxative stopped (unless being used for hepatic encephalopathy).
Monitoring	When treating inpatients, a stool chart is useful to monitor the effects of treatment. This is particularly important when treating hepatic encephalopathy, where you should also monitor electrolytes.
Cost	Osmotic laxatives are cheap. Patients who pay for their prescriptions may save money if they buy them over the counter.

Clinical tip—When treating faecal impaction with rectally administered laxatives, try a glycerol suppository (stimulant laxative) before using a phosphate enema. Glycerol suppositories are less likely to cause electrolyte disturbance. Phosphate enemas are irritant and are administered as a significant volume of fluid (>100 mL), which can be quite uncomfortable when administered. Reserve them for a second-line therapy.

Laxatives, stimulant

CLINICAL PHARMACOLOGY

Common indications	❶ **Constipation.** ❷ As suppositories for **faecal impaction.**
Mechanisms of action	Stimulant (also known as irritant or contact) laxatives **increase water and electrolyte secretion** from the colonic mucosa, thereby **increasing volume of colonic content and stimulating peristalsis.** They also have a direct pro-peristaltic action, although the exact mechanism differs between agents. For example, bacterial metabolism of senna in the intestine produces metabolites that have a direct action on the enteric nervous system, stimulating peristalsis. Rectal administration of stimulant laxatives, such as glycerol suppositories, provokes a similar but more localised effect and can be useful to treat faecal impaction. Docusate sodium has both stimulant and faecal softening actions.
Important adverse effects	Abdominal pain or cramping may occur with stimulant laxative use and diarrhoea is an obvious potential adverse effect. With prolonged use, some stimulant laxatives cause melanosis coli (reversible pigmentation of the intestinal wall).
Warnings	Stimulant laxatives should not be used in patients in whom ✖**intestinal obstruction** is suspected as there is a risk that this could induce **perforation.** Rectal preparations are usually avoided if ▲**haemorrhoids** or ▲**anal fissure** are present.
Important interactions	There are no clinically significant adverse drug interactions with stimulant laxatives.

senna, bisacodyl, glycerol suppositories, docusate sodium

PRACTICAL PRESCRIBING

Prescription	For **constipation,** you should generally prescribe stimulant laxatives for regular administration. They are usually taken twice a day and the dose is variable (e.g. 1–2 tablets of senna twice daily) and should be titrated to effect. When treating **faecal impaction,** rectal stimulant laxatives should usually be prescribed once only or as required with a maximum dose frequency of once in a 24-hour period.
Administration	Stimulant laxatives are usually administered orally, unless treating faecal impaction when glycerol suppositories may be administered rectally.
Communication	Explain that you are offering treatment with a laxative that will help stool to pass. As with other laxatives, ensuring good oral fluid intake will also help. Aim for 6–8 glasses of liquid per day. Advise your patient that stimulant laxatives do not work immediately and they may need a few doses before a sustained effect is noticed. Explain that the dose can be adjusted if necessary to maintain comfort. If they are regularly passing more than two or three soft stools per day, the dose should definitely be reduced or the laxative stopped. Mention that side effects such as abdominal cramps and flatulence can occur, but these may get better over time.
Monitoring	When treating inpatients, a stool chart is useful to monitor the effects of treatment.
Cost	Stimulant laxatives are cheap, around 10p a dose. Patients who pay for their prescriptions may save money if they buy them over the counter.

Clinical tip—When prescribing opioid analgesics to be taken regularly, consider co-prescribing a laxative to prevent constipation. A stimulant is a reasonable choice. Patients find constipation uncomfortable and it can contribute to confusion in the elderly, so prevention can increase adherence to opioid treatment and control of symptoms.

Lidocaine

CLINICAL PHARMACOLOGY

Common indications	❶ Very commonly, as a first choice **local anaesthetic** in, for example, **urinary catheterisation** and **minor procedures** (e.g. suturing). ❷ Uncommonly, as an antiarrhythmic drug in **ventricular tachycardia (VT)** and **ventricular fibrillation (VF) refractory to electrical cardioversion** (although <u>amiodarone</u> is preferred for the latter indication).
Mechanisms of action	Lidocaine (formerly known as lignocaine) enters cells in its uncharged form, then accepts a proton to become positively charged. From inside the cell, it enters and then **blocks voltage-gated sodium channels** on the surface membrane. This prevents initiation and propagation of action potentials in nerves and muscle, inducing local anaesthesia in the area supplied by blocked nerve fibres. In the heart, it reduces the duration of the action potential, slows conduction velocity and increases the refractory period. These effects may terminate VT and improve the chances of successfully treating VF.
Important adverse effects	The most common side effect is an initial **stinging** sensation during local administration. Systemic adverse effects are, predictably, more likely after systemic administration, whether intentional (as when it is used as an antiarrhythmic) or inadvertent (due to accidental intravascular injection during local administration). Its effects on the neurological system include **drowsiness, restlessness, tremor** and **fits.** It generally causes relatively little cardiovascular toxicity, but in overdose it may cause **hypotension** and **arrhythmias.**
Warnings	Used appropriately as a local anaesthetic, lidocaine is generally very safe. It depends heavily on hepatic blood flow for its elimination. Therefore, the dose should be reduced in states of ▲**reduced cardiac output.**
Important interactions	As the duration of action of local anaesthetics depends on how long they stay in contact with the neurones, co-administration with a vasoconstrictor (e.g. <u>adrenaline [epinephrine]</u>) produces a desirable interaction that may prolong the local anaesthetic effect.

lidocaine

PRACTICAL PRESCRIBING

Prescription	For **urinary catheterisation,** lidocaine is most commonly given as Instillagel®. This is a gel provided in pre-filled syringes. The dose is 6–11 mL. It *should* be prescribed in the once-only section, although in practice this is often omitted. For **minor procedures,** you usually use a 1% (10 mg/mL) solution of lidocaine hydrochloride. The maximum dose is 200 mg or 3 mg/kg, whichever is lower (7 mg/kg, or up to 500 mg, is permitted when it is combined with adrenaline). This should be calculated using *ideal body weight.* In practice, you draw up the dose you think you will need (ensuring this does not exceed the maximum), then administer enough to produce adequate anaesthesia. It is therefore acceptable to write the prescription and sign for its administration after completing the procedure. Foundation-level doctors should not prescribe lidocaine for systemic administration.
Administration	In **urinary catheterisation,** you open the packaging and allow the Instillagel® syringe to drop into your sterile field, ensuring asepsis is maintained. To administer it, you remove the cap, press the plunger gently to free it and expel any air, and then slowly inject the gel into the urethra. In **minor procedures,** you initially infiltrate the skin and superficial layers using a fine (orange) needle, then step up to a larger needle (blue or green) as necessary for deeper layers. Briefly retract the plunger before each injection to ensure you have not hit a vessel; this is signified by blood appearing in the syringe.
Communication	Explain that you are offering treatment with a local anaesthetic to numb the area before the procedure. Warn the patient that it will sting initially, but this will quickly disappear. They will still feel pushing and pulling sensations (from movement of surrounding non-anaesthetised tissues), but they should not feel pain. If they do, they should tell you.
Monitoring	Quality of anaesthesia is monitored clinically.
Cost	Lidocaine solution is cheap. Instillagel® costs about 10–20p per tube.

Clinical tip—A common mistake is not to wait long enough for lidocaine to reach maximal effect. There is no point infiltrating the area and then, 30 seconds later, repeatedly pricking the skin while saying 'can you feel this?' to the patient. They will feel it, and they will then lose confidence in your ability to deliver adequate anaesthesia. *Be patient.* Administer the local anaesthetic early, then turn back to your trolley and complete any necessary preparatory work. Try to wait a full 5 minutes before testing its effect.

Macrolides

CLINICAL PHARMACOLOGY

Common indications	❶ Treatment of **respiratory** and **skin and soft tissue infections** as an alternative to a <u>penicillin</u> when this is contraindicated by allergy. ❷ In **severe pneumonia** added to a penicillin to cover atypical organisms including *Legionella pneumophila* and *Mycoplasma pneumoniae*. ❸ Eradication of *Helicobacter pylori* (for example causing **peptic ulcer disease**) in combination with a <u>proton pump inhibitor</u> and either <u>amoxicillin</u> or <u>metronidazole</u>.
Mechanisms of action	Macrolides **inhibit bacterial protein synthesis.** They bind to the 50S subunit of the bacterial ribosome and block translocation, a process required for elongation of the polypeptide chain. Inhibition of protein synthesis is 'bacteriostatic' (stops bacteria growth), which assists the immune system in killing and removing bacteria from the body. Erythromycin, the first macrolide, was isolated from *Streptomycetes erythraeus* in the 1950s. It has a relatively broad spectrum of activity against Gram-positive and some Gram-negative organisms. Synthetic macrolides (e.g. clarithromycin and azithromycin) have increased activity against Gram-negative bacteria, particularly *Haemophilus influenzae*. Bacterial resistance to macrolides is common, mainly due to ribosomal mutations preventing macrolide binding.
Important adverse effects	Adverse effects are most common and severe with erythromycin, but can occur with any macrolide. Macrolides are **irritant,** causing nausea, vomiting, abdominal pain and diarrhoea when taken orally and thrombophlebitis when given IV. Other important side effects include **allergy, antibiotic-associated colitis** (see <u>Penicillins, broad-spectrum</u>), liver abnormalities including **cholestatic jaundice, prolongation of the QT interval** (predisposing to **arrhythmias**) and **ototoxicity** at high doses.
Warnings	Macrolides should not be prescribed if there is a history of ✖**macrolide hypersensitivity,** although they are a useful option where penicillin is contraindicated by allergy as there is no cross-sensitivity between these drug classes. Macrolide elimination from the body is mostly hepatic with a small renal contribution, such that caution is required in ▲**severe hepatic impairment** and dose reduction in ▲**severe renal impairment.**
Important interactions	Erythromycin and clarithromycin (but not azithromycin) inhibit cytochrome P450 enzymes. This increases plasma concentrations and risk of adverse effects with ▲**drugs metabolised by P450 enzymes.** For example, with <u>warfarin</u> there is an increased the risk of bleeding and with <u>statins</u> an increased risk of myopathy. Macrolides should be prescribed with caution in patients taking other ▲**drugs that prolong the QT interval** or cause arrhythmias, such as <u>amiodarone</u>, <u>antipsychotics</u>, <u>quinine</u>, <u>quinolone antibiotics</u> and <u>SSRIs</u>.

clarithromycin, erythromycin, azithromycin

PRACTICAL PRESCRIBING

Prescription	Clarithromycin is the most commonly prescribed macrolide in the UK, being more stable and causing fewer adverse effects than erythromycin, and being cheaper than azithromycin (which also is not formulated for IV administration). Clarithromycin is usually prescribed for oral administration, as it is absorbed readily in the intestine and has good bioavailability. It is prescribed IV where patients are unable to take or absorb drugs via the gastrointestinal tract (e.g. due to vomiting). The usual dosage is 250–500 mg twice daily for 7–14 days. When writing an inpatient antibiotic prescription, always include treatment indication and duration to facilitate good antibiotic stewardship.
Administration	Oral clarithromycin can be taken as tablets or oral suspension with or without food (although food may improve gastrointestinal tolerability). Intravenous clarithromycin should be diluted, e.g. 500 mg in 250 mL sodium chloride 0.9%, then infused into a large proximal vein (to reduce the risk of thrombophlebitis) over at least 60 minutes (to reduce the risk of arrhythmias). It must not be given as bolus IV or IM injection.
Communication	Explain that the aim of treatment is to get rid of infection and improve symptoms. For oral treatment, encourage the patient to complete the prescribed course. Before prescribing, always check with your patient personally or get collateral history to ensure that they are not allergic to macrolides. Warn them to seek medical advice if a rash or other unexpected symptoms develop. If an allergy develops during treatment, give the patient written and verbal advice not to take this antibiotic in the future and make sure that the allergy is clearly documented in their medical records.
Monitoring	Check that infection resolves by patient report (e.g. resolution of symptoms), examination (e.g. resolution of pyrexia, lung crackles) and blood tests (e.g. falling C-reactive protein and white cell count), as appropriate.
Cost	Where IV clarithromycin is prescribed, switch to oral as soon as tolerated as this reduces the cost of the drug (IV around £9.50/day, oral around 50p/day), administration costs, complications and inpatient stay.

Clinical tip—In patients with lower respiratory tract infections (LRTI), macrolides should generally only be added to penicillin treatment if there is **evidence of pneumonia** (e.g. consolidation on the chest X-ray). Macrolides are required to cover penicillin-resistant atypical organisms, e.g. *Legionella pneumophila* and *Mycoplasma pneumoniae*, that cause pneumonia but do not cause other LRTI, e.g. COPD exacerbations.

Metformin

CLINICAL PHARMACOLOGY

Common indications	❶ **Type 2 diabetes mellitus,** as first choice medication for control of blood glucose, used alone or in combination with other oral hypoglycaemic drugs (e.g. <u>sulphonylureas</u>) or <u>insulin</u>.
Mechanisms of action	Metformin (a biguanide) lowers blood glucose by **increasing the response (sensitivity) to insulin.** It suppresses hepatic glucose production (glycogenolysis and gluconeogenesis), increases glucose uptake and utilisation by skeletal muscle and suppresses intestinal glucose absorption. It achieves this by diverse intracellular mechanisms, which are incompletely understood. It does not stimulate pancreatic insulin secretion and therefore does not cause hypoglycaemia. It **reduces weight gain** and can induce weight loss, which can prevent worsening of insulin resistance and slow deterioration of diabetes mellitus.
Important adverse effects	Metformin commonly causes **gastrointestinal upset,** including nausea, vomiting, taste disturbance, anorexia and diarrhoea. This adverse effect may contribute to weight loss in patients taking metformin. **Lactic acidosis** is a rare adverse effect associated with metformin use, which can be fatal if untreated. It does not occur in stable patients, but can be precipitated by intercurrent illness that causes metformin accumulation (e.g. worsening renal impairment), increased lactate production (e.g. sepsis, hypoxia, cardiac failure) or reduced lactate metabolism (e.g. liver failure).
Warnings	Metformin is excreted unchanged by the kidney. Metformin is therefore contraindicated in ✖**severe renal impairment** and a dose reduction is required for patients with ▲**moderate renal impairment.** Metformin should be withheld acutely where there is ✖**acute kidney injury,** e.g. in sepsis, shock, or dehydration; or ✖**severe tissue hypoxia,** e.g. in cardiac or respiratory failure, or myocardial infarction. Caution is required in ▲**hepatic impairment** as clearance of excess lactate may be impaired. Metformin should be withheld during ▲**acute alcohol intoxication**, when it may precipitate lactic acidosis, and be used with caution in ▲**chronic alcohol overuse,** where there is a risk of hypoglycaemia.
Important interactions	Metformin must be withheld before and for 48 hours after injection of ▲**IV contrast media** (e.g. for CT scans, coronary angiography) when there is an increased risk of renal impairment, metformin accumulation and lactic acidosis. Other drugs (e.g. <u>ACE inhibitors</u>, <u>NSAIDs</u>, <u>diuretics</u>) with potential to impair renal function should also be used with caution (e.g. with renal function monitoring) in combination with metformin. <u>Prednisolone</u>, <u>thiazide</u> and <u>loop diuretics</u> elevate blood glucose, hence oppose the actions and reduce efficacy of metformin.

PRACTICAL PRESCRIBING

Prescription	Metformin is only available for **oral administration.** Gastrointestinal adverse effects of metformin are usually transient and are best tolerated if metformin is started at a **low dose** and **increased gradually.** A common regimen is to start metformin 500 mg once daily with breakfast, increasing the dose by 500 mg weekly to 500–850 mg three times daily with meals. Metformin is a **long-term** treatment that in general should only be stopped or changed if adverse effects are intolerable or new contraindications develop.
Administration	Patients should be started on a standard-release preparation of metformin and advised to swallow tablets whole with a glass of water **with or after food.** If gastrointestinal effects are intolerable, changing from standard to a modified-release preparation may help.
Communication	Advise patients that metformin has been prescribed to control the blood sugar level and reduce the risk of diabetic complications, such as heart attacks. Explain that tablets are not a replacement for **lifestyle measures** and should be taken in addition to a calorie-controlled diet and regular exercise. Warn them to seek **urgent medical advice** if they experience vomiting, stomach ache, muscle cramps, difficulty breathing or severe tiredness, which may be symptoms of a very rare side effect called **lactic acidosis.** Advise them always to tell a doctor that they are taking metformin before having an **X-ray or operation,** as metformin may need to be stopped before the procedure.
Monitoring	Assess blood glucose control by measuring **glycated haemoglobin (HbA$_{1c}$)** (target <58 mmol/mol). Blood glucose monitoring is not routinely required. For **safety,** measure renal function before starting treatment, then at least annually. Renal function should be measured more frequently (at least twice per year) in people with deteriorating renal function or at increased risk of renal impairment.
Cost	Non-proprietary metformin 500 mg tablets cost around 1p each. More complicated formulations (e.g. oral solution, modified release, combinations with other oral hypoglycaemics) are more expensive.

Clinical tip—Increasing body weight increases insulin resistance, which can cause or worsen type 2 diabetes mellitus. Initial treatment for type 2 diabetes mellitus is therefore calorie and carbohydrate restriction with increased physical activity, which should be tried for at least 3 months before commencing drug therapy. As insulin is an anabolic hormone, it and drugs which increase insulin secretion (e.g. sulphonylureas) cause weight gain, which can worsen diabetes mellitus over the long term. Metformin, which does not cause weight gain, is therefore usually the first choice treatment unless contraindicated.

Methotrexate

CLINICAL PHARMACOLOGY

Common indications	❶ As a disease-modifying treatment for **rheumatoid arthritis.** ❷ As part of **chemotherapy** regimens for cancers including **leukaemia**, **lymphoma** and some **solid tumours.** ❸ To treat severe **psoriasis** (including **psoriatic arthritis)** that is resistant to other therapies.
Mechanisms of action	Methotrexate **inhibits dihydrofolate reductase,** which converts dietary folic acid to tetrahydrofolate (FH4). FH4 is required for DNA and protein synthesis, so lack of FH4 **prevents cellular replication.** Actively dividing cells are particularly sensitive to the effects of methotrexate, accounting for its efficacy in **cancer.** Methotrexate also has anti-inflammatory and immunosuppressive effects. These are mediated in part by inhibition of inflammatory mediators such as interleukin (IL)-6, IL-8 and tumour necrosis factor (TNF)-α, although the underlying mechanisms are not fully understood.
Important adverse effects	Dose-related adverse effects of methotrexate include **mucosal damage** (e.g. sore mouth, gastrointestinal upset) and **bone marrow suppression** (resulting most significantly in neutropenia and an increased risk of infection). Rarely, **hypersensitivity reactions** including cutaneous reactions, hepatitis or pneumonitis may occur. Long-term use can cause **hepatic cirrhosis** or **pulmonary fibrosis.** As methotrexate is usually administered once weekly (see Prescription), there is a risk of accidental **overdose** if patients take treatment daily. Overdose causes severe dose-related adverse effects with renal impairment and hepatotoxicity. Neurological effects such as headache, seizures and coma may also occur. Treatment is with folinic acid, which 'rescues' normal cells from methotrexate effects, and with hydration and urinary alkalinisation to enhance methotrexate excretion.
Warnings	Methotrexate is **teratogenic** and must be avoided in ✖**pregnancy.** Both men and women taking the drug should use effective contraception during and for 3 months after stopping treatment. As methotrexate is renally excreted, it is contraindicated in ✖**severe renal impairment.** As it can cause hepatotoxicity, methotrexate should be avoided in ▲**abnormal liver function.**
Important interactions	Methotrexate toxicity is more likely if it is prescribed with drugs that inhibit its renal excretion, e.g. ▲NSAIDs, ▲penicillins. Co-prescription with ▲**other folate antagonists,** e.g. trimethoprim and phenytoin, increases the risk of haematological abnormalities. The risk of neutropenia is increased if methotrexate is combined with ▲clozapine.

PRACTICAL PRESCRIBING

Prescription	For **autoimmune disease,** methotrexate is prescribed for oral administration. A typical dose would be 7.5–20 mg **once weekly,** adjusted according to response and adverse effects (which are more common at higher doses). It is crucial to emphasise the once weekly nature of this prescription. Folic acid 5 mg can be prescribed to be taken on the 6 days where methotrexate is not taken. This may limit adverse effects. For **cancer,** methotrexate may be given by IV, IM or intrathecal routes to induce remission, then orally for maintenance treatment. Treatment for this indication should be by specialists only.
Administration	**Intravenous** and **intrathecal administration** of methotrexate should be done only by healthcare practitioners who have had sufficient training and in carefully regulated circumstances.
Communication	Explain that methotrexate treatment should cause improvement in, for example, swollen painful joints, but that this may take some time to reach maximal effect. Emphasise that methotrexate should be **taken once a week** (not every day) by prompting the patient to consider on what day they will take it. Warn patients to seek urgent medical advice if they develop sore throat or fever (infection), bruising or bleeding (low platelet count), nausea, abdominal pain or dark urine (liver poisoning) or breathlessness (lung toxicity). Give advice regarding contraception (see Warnings) to all patients (men and women) who have potential to have a child.
Monitoring	**Efficacy** should be monitored by symptoms, examination (e.g. of inflamed joints) and blood tests (e.g. inflammatory markers). **Safety** monitoring is essential as adverse effects can be life threatening, but may be reversible if detected early and treatment is stopped. Patients should be advised to report unexpected symptoms (see above). Measure full blood count, liver and renal function before starting treatment, then 1–2 weekly until treatment is established and 2–3 monthly thereafter. Treatment should be stopped immediately if abnormalities develop or if the patient becomes breathless.
Cost	Non-proprietary oral methotrexate is available and is inexpensive.

Clinical tip—There are significant restrictions associated with the prescription of methotrexate in order to reduce medication errors and the risk of toxicity. Foundation year 1 doctors **should not** initiate a methotrexate prescription. They may have an important role in reviewing or continuing prescriptions, for example at the time of hospital admission. If in any doubt about the appropriateness of a methotrexate prescription, always seek senior advice.

Metronidazole

CLINICAL PHARMACOLOGY

Common indications	Treatment of infections caused by anaerobic bacteria in: ❶ **Antibiotic-associated colitis** caused by *Clostridium difficile,* which is a Gram-positive anaerobe. ❷ **Oral infections** (such as dental abscess) or **aspiration pneumonia** caused by Gram-negative anaerobes from the mouth. ❸ **Surgical and gynaecological infections** caused by Gram-negative anaerobes from the colon, for example *Bacteroides fragilis.* ❹ Also effective for treatment of **protozoal infections** including trichomonal vaginal infection, amoebic dysentery, giardiasis.
Mechanisms of action	Metronidazole enters bacterial cells by passive diffusion. In **anaerobic bacteria,** reduction of metronidazole generates a nitroso free radical. This binds to DNA, reducing synthesis and causing widespread damage, **DNA degradation** and **cell death.** As aerobic bacteria are not able to reduce metronidazole in this manner, the spectrum of action of metronidazole is restricted to anaerobic bacteria (and protozoa). Bacterial resistance to metronidazole is generally low but is increasing in prevalence. Mechanisms include reduced uptake of metronidazole and reduced generation of nitroso free radicals.
Important adverse effects	As with many antibiotics, metronidazole can cause **gastrointestinal upset** (such as nausea and vomiting) and immediate and delayed **hypersensitivity** reactions (see <u>Penicillins, broad-spectrum</u>). When used at high doses or for a prolonged course, metronidazole can cause neurological adverse effects including **peripheral** and **optic neuropathy, seizures** and **encephalopathy.**
Warnings	Metronidazole is metabolised by hepatic cytochrome P450 enzymes, so the dose should be reduced in people with ▲**severe liver disease.** Metronidazole inhibits the enzyme acetaldehyde dehydrogenase, which is responsible for clearing the intermediate alcohol metabolite acetaldehyde from the body. ✖**Alcohol** should not be drunk while taking metronidazole as the combination can cause a 'disulfiram-like' reaction, including flushing, headache, nausea and vomiting.
Important interactions	Metronidazole has some inhibitory effect on **cytochrome P450 enzymes,** reducing metabolism of <u>warfarin</u> (increasing the risk of bleeding) and <u>phenytoin</u> (increasing the risk of toxicity, including impaired cerebellar function). The reverse interaction can occur with ▲**cytochrome P450 inducers** (e.g. <u>phenytoin</u>, rifampicin) resulting in reduced plasma concentrations and impaired antimicrobial efficacy. Metronidazole also increases the risk of toxicity with lithium.

PRACTICAL PRESCRIBING

Prescription	Metronidazole is available in a variety of formulations. The oral route is used for gastrointestinal infection or where the patient is not systemically unwell. A typical starting dose would be 400 mg orally 8-hrly. The intravenous route, usually at a dose of 500 mg IV 8-hrly, is used for severe infection or where patients cannot take treatment by mouth. Rectal metronidazole is an alternative for patients who are nil by mouth. Metronidazole can be prescribed as a gel for topical administration to treat vaginal infection such as bacterial vaginosis or to reduce the odour from an infected skin ulcer.
Administration	Oral metronidazole may be taken as tablets or in an oral suspension. Intravenous metronidazole is given as an infusion over 20 minutes.
Communication	Explain that the aim of treatment is to get rid of infection and improve symptoms. For oral treatment, encourage the patient to complete the prescribed course. Before prescribing, always check with your patient personally or get collateral history to ensure that they have no **allergy** to metronidazole. Warn the patient not to take **alcohol** during or for 48 hours after treatment, explaining that if they do they may feel very unwell with nausea, vomiting, flushing and headache. If an allergy develops during treatment, give the patient written and verbal advice not to take this antibiotic in the future and make sure that the allergy is clearly documented in their medical records.
Monitoring	Check that infection resolves by review of symptoms, signs and blood tests (improvement in inflammatory markers) if appropriate. For treatment exceeding 10 days, measure full blood count and liver function tests to monitor for adverse effects.
Cost	A 7-day course of non-proprietary oral metronidazole tablets taken one 8-hrly currently costs around £1.50 if 400 mg tablets are prescribed, but around £36 if 500 mg tablets are prescribed. You should therefore select the lower dose unless there are overwhelming clinical indications for the higher dose.

Clinical tip—Anaerobic bacteria are often resistant to penicillins due to production of β-lactamases. However, co-amoxiclav (amoxicillin with the β-lactamase inhibitor clavulanic acid) does have good efficacy against anaerobes. Where patients are taking co-amoxiclav (e.g. for aspiration pneumonia) anaerobic cover is often sufficient and there is no need to add metronidazole. However, you should consult local antibiotic guidelines and seek microbiology advice to support prescribing, particularly if your patient does not improve with first-line treatment.

Naloxone

CLINICAL PHARMACOLOGY

Common indications	❶ Treatment of **opioid toxicity** associated with respiratory and/or neurological depression.
Mechanisms of action	Naloxone binds to opioid receptors (particularly the pharmacologically-important opioid μ-receptors), where it acts as a **competitive antagonist.** It has little or no effect in the absence of an exogenous opioid (e.g. morphine). However, if an opioid is present, naloxone displaces it from its receptors and, in so doing, it reverses its effects. In opioid toxicity, this is used to restore an adequate level of consciousness and respiratory rate.
Important adverse effects	Where naloxone is administered to reverse opioid toxicity in an opioid-dependent individual, an **opioid withdrawal reaction** may be precipitated. This presents with pain (if the opioid was being taken for its analgesic effect), restlessness, nausea and vomiting, dilated pupils, and cold, dry skin with piloerection ('cold turkey'). Naloxone has no other significant adverse effects.
Warnings	There are no specific contraindications to the use of naloxone. However, caution should be exercised in patients who may have developed ▲**opioid dependence** (whether from therapeutic or recreational use) because of the risk of precipitating opioid withdrawal. Lower doses should be used in the ▲**palliative care** setting to reduce the risk of complete reversal of analgesia.
Important interactions	Naloxone has no clinically important drug interactions other than its interaction with opioids, which is central to its pharmacological effect and practical use.

naloxone

PRACTICAL PRESCRIBING

Prescription	Acute opioid toxicity can usually be adequately reversed with naloxone 400–1200 micrograms IV, titrated to effect (see Administration). If IV access is inappropriate or unavailable, it can be given IM, SC, or intranasally. It is best to prescribe naloxone in the once-only section of the drug chart. As it is often given by a physician in an emergency setting, the prescription may be written at the time of administration, or immediately after.
Administration	Naloxone is usually administered by the prescriber or under their direct supervision. It should be given in small incremental doses (typically 200–400 micrograms IV) every 2–3 minutes, until satisfactory reversal is achieved (patient rousable with adequate respiratory rate). In patients who develop opioid toxicity in the context of chronic use (especially in palliative care), smaller incremental doses (40–100 micrograms) should be used.
Communication	Once opioid toxicity has been reversed and the patient is awake, you can, as appropriate, explain that they were given an antidote to counteract the effect of having too much morphine (for example) in their body. Depending on the clinical context, you may need to discuss how this situation arose and how to avoid it in future.
Monitoring	Patients should be **closely monitored** during naloxone administration, as the dose is titrated to effect. Once adequate reversal is achieved, it is essential to continue monitoring for at least an hour. This is because the duration of action of naloxone (about 20–60 min, depending on route of administration) is shorter than that of most opioids. Consequently, **opioid toxicity can recur** when the effect of naloxone has dissipated, necessitating repeated doses or, occasionally, an infusion.
Cost	Naloxone is available in non-proprietary form and is inexpensive.

Clinical tip—When giving small doses of naloxone (e.g. 40 micrograms, which may be used in a palliative care setting), it is impractical to use the 400 microgram/mL solution that is usually provided in hospitals. Therefore, take 1 mL (400 micrograms) of this solution and mix it in a syringe with 9 mL of 0.9% sodium chloride. This will result in a 40 microgram/mL solution, which you can then administer in more practical 1 mL increments. Ensure the syringe is clearly labelled with details of its contents.

Nicorandil

CLINICAL PHARMACOLOGY

Common indications	❶ For prevention and treatment of chest pain in people with **stable angina.** First choice treatments for stable angina are β-blockers and calcium channel blockers, individually or in combination. Nicorandil (or a long-acting nitrate) may be used if these drugs are insufficient or not tolerated.
Mechanisms of action	Nicorandil causes both arterial and venous vasodilatation through its **actions as a nitrate** (see Nitrates) and by **activating K⁺-ATP channels.** Efflux of K⁺ through activated K⁺-ATP channels leads to hyperpolarisation of the cell membrane and subsequent inactivation of voltage-gated Ca^{2+} channels. The net effect is a decrease in free intracellular calcium. As calcium is required for smooth muscle contraction, relaxation and **vasodilatation** occur. The effect of this is to reduce cardiac preload and systemic and coronary vascular resistance. This **improves myocardial perfusion,** and **decreases myocardial work** and **oxygen demand.** Clinically, this reduces the frequency and severity of angina attacks.
Important adverse effects	Unwanted effects of vasodilatation include **flushing, dizziness** and **headache.** Nicorandil can also cause **nausea, vomiting** and **hypotension.** Less frequently, it can cause **gastrointestinal, skin or mucosal ulceration,** which only responds to withdrawal of treatment.
Warnings	You should not routinely prescribe nicorandil for patients with ▲**poor left ventricular function,** ▲**hypotension** or ▲**pulmonary oedema,** as it can worsen these conditions.
Important interactions	As with nitrates, the hypotensive side effects of nicorandil are significantly enhanced by ✖phosphodiesterase inhibitors (e.g. sildenafil). They should not be prescribed together.

PRACTICAL PRESCRIBING

Prescription	Nicorandil is only available for oral administration. It is started at a low dose of 5–10 mg twice daily and increased to 20–30 mg twice daily as the patient becomes tolerant of the vasodilatory adverse effects.
Administration	Oral nicorandil is formulated as tablets without other options for administration.
Communication	Advise the patient that nicorandil has been prescribed to **reduce attacks of chest pain.** Explain that they should take the treatment for the foreseeable future. Discuss other measures to **reduce cardiovascular risk,** including smoking cessation. Warn patients **not to drive or use heavy machinery** until angina symptoms are controlled and side effects of nicorandil, including dizziness and hypotension, have settled.
Monitoring	You should review angina symptoms on a regular basis and increase the dose of nicorandil to the maximum tolerated. Blood pressure should be measured to check for hypotension.
Cost	Prescribe nicorandil using its generic name as this will allow the pharmacist to dispense the non-proprietary formulation rather than the branded preparation, which is about twice as expensive.

Clinical tip—Patients whose symptoms are not controlled on two anti-anginal drugs need to be referred to a cardiologist for review and consideration of angiography and revascularisation. Requirement for nicorandil treatment could therefore be considered as a trigger for cardiology referral.

Nicotine replacement and related drugs

CLINICAL PHARMACOLOGY

Common indications	❶ In **smoking cessation,** drug therapy to control physical symptoms of nicotine withdrawal is used alongside non-pharmacological measures to address the psychological and behavioural aspects of dependence.
Mechanisms of action	Nicotine obtained from tobacco use has complex actions. In the central nervous system it **activates nicotinic acetylcholine receptors,** increasing neurotransmitter levels and causing euphoria and relaxation. Nicotine withdrawal causes intense craving, anxiety, depression and irritability with increased appetite and weight gain. During abstinence from tobacco, *nicotine replacement therapy* **prevents withdrawal symptoms** by maintaining receptor activation. *Varenicline*, a partial agonist of the nicotinic receptor, reduces both withdrawal symptoms and the rewarding effects of smoking by preventing binding of tobacco-derived nicotine to receptors. *Bupropion* increases concentrations of noradrenaline and dopamine in the synaptic cleft by inhibiting reuptake. The mechanism underlying its benefits in smoking cessation are not fully understood.
Important adverse effects	It is generally considered safer for smokers to take nicotine replacement therapy than to continue smoking. Adverse effects include **local irritation** (for example from patches, lozenges, nasal spray) or **gastrointestinal upset** with oral nicotine. Palpitations and abnormal dreams may occur. Common side effects of *varenicline* include nausea, headache, insomnia and abnormal dreams. Rarely, patients may develop **suicidal ideation.** *Bupropion* commonly causes **dry mouth, gastrointestinal upset, neurological** (e.g. headache, impaired concentration, dizziness) and **psychiatric** (e.g. insomnia, depression, agitation) adverse effects. Hypersensitivity is common and more often manifests as a skin rash (for example urticaria) than a severe reaction (such as anaphylaxis).
Warnings	*Nicotine replacement therapy* should be used with caution in people who are ▲**haemodynamically unstable,** for example following myocardial infarction. *Bupropion* and *varenicline* should be used with caution in people ▲**at risk of seizures** as they can precipitate convulsions. This includes people with prior seizures or head injury and those who abuse alcohol or who take other drugs that lower the seizure threshold. They should be used with care in people with ▲**psychiatric disease** due to risk of suicidal ideation. All these drugs should be used with caution in people with ▲**hepatic** or **renal impairment.**
Important interactions	*Nicotine replacement* and *varenicline* have no clinically significant drug interactions. *Bupropion* is metabolised by cytochrome P450 enzymes, so its plasma levels are increased by ▲**P450 inhibitors,** e.g. valproate, and reduced by **inducers,** e.g. phenytoin, carbamazepine. Use of bupropion with monoamine oxidase inhibitors or tricyclic antidepressants increases stimulation of catecholaminergic pathways and risk of adverse effects.

PRACTICAL PRESCRIBING

Prescription	*Nicotine replacement therapy* is prescribed as a **continuous-release patch** to reduce or prevent cravings and/or an **immediate-release preparation** (for example sublingual tablets, sprays, gum) to control the acute urge to smoke. Treatment should start either before a cessation attempt to reduce the number of cigarettes smoked or when the patient stops smoking. For people smoking >10 cigarettes/day, start treatment with a high-dose nicotine patch for 6–8 weeks, then wean to a medium then low-dose patch for 2 weeks each before stopping. Treatment with *varenicline* or *bupropion* should start 1–2 weeks before the target quit date. A low starting dose is titrated over the first week to the optimal treatment dose and continued for 9–12 weeks. The drug is stopped if the smoking cessation attempt fails.
Administration	**Nicotine patches** should be applied in the morning to an area of dry hairless skin and taken off at night to prevent insomnia. They should be applied to a different site each day to reduce skin irritation. **Immediate-release nicotine** in any formulation should be taken as soon as the urge to smoke strikes.
Communication	Explain that the medicine offered can help to **reduce the craving** for a cigarette and the feeling of irritability that can occur when stopping smoking. Advise them that treatment works best if they have a plan as to how and when they will stop and have thought about how they might change their habits to stay off cigarettes. Offer **support and counselling,** for example through a smoking cessation clinic, as this increases the chance of a successful quit attempt.
Monitoring	Monitoring the success of a quit attempt and side effects of treatment is usually by **patient report.** Patients should be reviewed monthly, for example as part of a smoking cessation clinic.
Cost	Drugs to help with smoking cessation can be **prescribed on the NHS,** but only for patients who have a clear idea of how and when they will quit. A course of any treatment to support smoking cessation (10–12 weeks) costs approximately £150. Treatment should therefore be stopped if the attempt fails and should not usually be repeated within 6 months, unless exceptional circumstances have interrupted the attempt.

Clinical tip—Acute hospital admission causes anxiety and immobility, both of which can encourage people to stop smoking. Ask all inpatients about smoking and offer nicotine replacement as patches and/or immediate-release preparations to current smokers. Refer those interested to smoking cessation services for ongoing support on discharge.

Nitrates

CLINICAL PHARMACOLOGY

Common indications	❶ Short-acting nitrates (glyceryl trinitrate) are used in the treatment of **acute angina** and chest pain associated with **acute coronary syndrome.** ❷ Long-acting nitrates (e.g. isosorbide mononitrate) are used for **prophylaxis of angina** where a β-blocker and/or a calcium channel blocker are insufficient or not tolerated. ❸ Intravenous nitrates are used in the treatment of **pulmonary oedema,** usually in combination with furosemide and oxygen.
Mechanisms of action	Nitrates are converted to nitric oxide (NO). NO increases cyclic guanosine monophosphate (cGMP) synthesis and reduces intracellular Ca^{2+} in vascular smooth muscle cells, causing them to relax. This results in venous and, to a lesser extent, arterial vasodilatation. **Relaxation of the venous capacitance vessels** reduces cardiac preload and left ventricular filling. These effects **reduce cardiac work and myocardial oxygen demand,** relieving angina and cardiac failure. Nitrates can relieve coronary vasospasm and dilate collateral vessels, improving coronary perfusion. They also relax the systemic arteries, reducing peripheral resistance and afterload. However, most of the anti-anginal effects are mediated by reduction of preload.
Important adverse effects	As vasodilators, nitrates commonly cause **flushing, headaches, light-headedness** and **hypotension.** Sustained use of nitrates can lead to **tolerance,** with reduced symptom relief despite continued use. This can be minimised by careful timing of doses to avoid significant nitrate exposure overnight, when it tends not to be needed.
Warnings	Nitrates are contraindicated in patients with ✖**severe aortic stenosis,** in whom they may cause cardiovascular collapse. This is because the heart is unable to increase cardiac output sufficiently through the narrowed valve area to maintain pressure in the now dilated vasculature. Nitrates should also be avoided in patients with ✖**haemodynamic instability,** particularly ✖**hypotension.**
Important interactions	Nitrates must not be used with ✖phosphodiesterase inhibitors (e.g. sildenafil) because these enhance and prolong the hypotensive effect of nitrates. Nitrates should also be used with caution in patients taking antihypertensive medication, in whom they may precipitate hypotension.

isosorbide mononitrate, glyceryl trinitrate

PRACTICAL PRESCRIBING

Prescription	In patients with **stable angina,** glyceryl trinitrate (GTN) is prescribed to be taken **sublingually** as tablets or spray for immediate relief of chest pain. GTN has a plasma half-life of <5 minutes, so has a very quick onset and offset of action. In patients with **acute coronary syndrome** or **heart failure,** GTN is prescribed as a **continuous intravenous infusion.** Isosorbide mononitrate (ISMN) has a plasma half-life of 4–5 hours and is prescribed two to three times daily as immediate-release **tablets** for the prevention of recurrent angina. ISMN is also available as modified-release tablets or transdermal **patches,** which are prescribed once daily. When prescribing modified-release preparations, prescribe by the brand name, since there are important differences between preparations.
Administration	IV GTN is usually administered as a solution containing GTN 50 mg in 50 mL (1 mg/mL). You should give nursing staff clear instructions on the starting dose, normally expressed as an infusion rate, e.g. 1 mL/hr. You should provide instructions on how to increase the dose to relieve symptoms (e.g. 'Increase GTN infusion rate by 0.5 mL/hr every 15–30 minutes until chest pain relieved') while avoiding hypotension (e.g. 'Keep systolic blood pressure >90 mmHg').
Communication	Explain that you are prescribing a nitrate to relieve chest pain and/or breathlessness. Advise your patient that they may develop a headache when starting nitrates, but that this is normally short-lived. As nitrates are probably more effective at preventing than terminating angina, patients should be advised to use sublingual GTN *before* tasks that normally bring on their angina. Due to the risks of postural hypotension, it is a good idea to advise them to sit down and rest before and for 5 minutes after taking sublingual GTN.
Monitoring	The best indicators of efficacy are the patient's **symptoms** (e.g. chest pain, breathlessness). When administering nitrates by IV infusion, **blood pressure** should be monitored frequently, and the infusion rate adjusted to ensure the systolic blood pressure does not drop below 90 mmHg.
Cost	Non-proprietary GTN and isosorbide mononitrate are inexpensive. GTN sublingual tablets must be discarded after 8 weeks, so a spray may be a better choice for patients with infrequent symptoms.

Clinical tip—Where nitrates are taken regularly, there is a risk of tolerance (tachyphylaxis), which can reduce efficacy. To prevent this, time doses to ensure there is a 'nitrate-free period' every day during a time of inactivity, usually overnight. For example, patients should be advised to take twice daily isosorbide mononitrate morning and mid-afternoon (rather than evening) to ensure >12 hours between pm and am doses. Transdermal patches should be applied in the morning and removed at bedtime.

Nitrofurantoin

CLINICAL PHARMACOLOGY

Common indications	❶ **Uncomplicated lower urinary tract infection (UTI),** as a first-line antibiotic (alternatives are <u>trimethoprim</u>, <u>amoxicillin</u>). Nitrofurantoin is particularly suited to the treatment of UTI as it is effective against the common causative organisms, reaches therapeutic concentrations in urine through renal excretion, and is most bactericidal in acidic environments such as urine.
Mechanisms of action	Nitrofurantoin is metabolised (reduced) in bacterial cells by nitrofuran reductase. Its **active metabolite damages bacterial DNA** and causes cell death (bactericidal effect). Nitrofurantoin is active against the Gram-negative (e.g. *Escherichia coli*) and Gram-positive (*Staphylococcus saprophyticus*) organisms that commonly cause urinary tract infections. Bacteria with reduced nitrofuran reductase activity are resistant to nitrofurantoin. Some organisms that are less common causes of urinary tract infection (such as klebsiella and proteus species) have intrinsic resistance to nitrofurantoin. It is relatively rare for *E. coli* to acquire nitrofurantoin resistance.
Important adverse effects	As with many antibiotics, nitrofurantoin can cause **gastrointestinal upset** (including nausea and diarrhoea) and immediate and delayed **hypersensitivity** reactions (see <u>Penicillins, broad-spectrum</u>). Nitrofurantoin specifically can turn urine dark yellow or brown. Less commonly, it may cause **chronic pulmonary reactions** (including inflammation [pneumonitis] and fibrosis), **hepatitis** and **peripheral neuropathy,** which all are more likely with prolonged administration. In neonates, **haemolytic anaemia** may occur because immature red blood cells are unable to mop up nitrofurantoin-stimulated superoxides, which damage red blood cells.
Warnings	Nitrofurantoin should not be prescribed for ✖**pregnant women towards term** or for ✖**babies in the first 3 months of life.** It is contraindicated in patients with ✖**renal impairment**, as impaired excretion increases toxicity and reduces efficacy due to lower urinary drug concentrations. Caution is required when using nitrofurantoin for ▲**long-term prevention** of UTIs, as chronic use increases the risk of adverse effects, particularly in elderly patients.
Important interactions	There are no significant interactions between nitrofurantoin and other commonly prescribed drugs.

PRACTICAL PRESCRIBING

Prescription	Nitrofurantoin is only available for oral administration. Maximum urinary concentrations are usually achieved 2–4 hours after dosing.

For **treatment of acute UTI,** a typical dosage regimen is 50–100 mg 6-hrly. Treatment duration depends on nature and severity of infection, with a 3-day course being sufficient for uncomplicated UTIs in women and 7 days of treatment being required for men or for more complicated infection.

For **prevention of recurrent UTI,** a single nightly dose of 50–100 mg is prescribed. Treatment duration should only be longer than 6 months if strongly indicated, and this requires monitoring (see below). |
Administration	Oral nitrofurantoin is available as tablets, capsules and in suspension. It should be **taken with food or milk** to minimise gastrointestinal effects.
Communication	Explain that the aim of treatment is to get rid of infection and improve symptoms. Encourage the patient to complete the prescribed course. Before prescribing, always check with your patient personally or get collateral history to ensure that they do not have an **allergy** to nitrofurantoin. Advise them that their **urine colour** may change to dark yellow or brown during treatment; this is harmless and temporary. In long-term treatment, warn patients to report any unexplained symptoms, particularly **pins and needles** or **breathlessness,** which could indicate serious side effects.
Monitoring	Efficacy of **treatment for acute UTI** is determined by resolution of symptoms and, less commonly, by ensuring sterility of urine on repeat culture. Success in **preventing recurrent UTI** is determined by comparing UTI frequency before and during prophylaxis. Safety of long-term treatment is a particular concern and patients should be advised to report any symptoms (see Communication) that could indicate the onset of neuropathy or pulmonary adverse effects.
Cost	Costs of a 7-day course of nitrofurantoin 50 mg 6-hrly vary widely between preparations (£4 to £170 for a 1-week course). However, if you prescribe nitrofurantoin using the non-proprietary name, the pharmacist is able to dispense the cheapest formulation available.

Clinical tip—As tissue concentrations of nitrofurantoin are very low, you should not prescribe it for pyelonephritis or other complicated urinary tract infections. A suitable alternative regimen for these indications would be co-amoxiclav with gentamicin.

Non-steroidal anti-inflammatory drugs

CLINICAL PHARMACOLOGY

Common indications	❶ 'As needed' treatment of **mild-to-moderate pain** (e.g. dysmenorrhoea, dental pain) as an alternative to or in addition to <u>paracetamol</u>. Analgesia from a single dose of a non-steroidal anti-inflammatory drug (NSAID) is similar to that from paracetamol, which is therefore preferred, particularly in those at risk of adverse effects. ❷ Regular treatment for **pain related to inflammation,** particularly of the musculoskeletal system, e.g. in rheumatoid arthritis, severe osteoarthritis and acute gout.
Mechanisms of action	NSAIDs inhibit synthesis of prostaglandins from arachidonic acid by **inhibiting cyclooxygenase** (COX). COX exists as two main isoforms. COX-1 is the *constitutive* form. It stimulates prostaglandin synthesis that is essential to preserve integrity of the gastric mucosa; maintain renal perfusion (by dilating afferent glomerular arterioles); and inhibit thrombus formation at the vascular endothelium. COX-2 is the *inducible* form, expressed in response to inflammatory stimuli. It stimulates production of prostaglandins that cause inflammation and pain. The therapeutic benefits of NSAIDs are principally mediated by COX-2 inhibition and adverse effects by COX-1 inhibition, although there is some overlap between the two. Selective COX-2 inhibitors (e.g. etoricoxib) were developed in an attempt to reduce the adverse effects of NSAIDs.
Important adverse effects	The main adverse effects of NSAIDs are **gastrointestinal (GI) toxicity, renal impairment** and increased risk of **cardiovascular (CV) events** (e.g. myocardial infarction and stroke). The likelihood of adverse effects differs between NSAIDs. Of all the non-selective NSAIDs (>20 are available), ibuprofen is associated with the lowest risk of GI effects. Naproxen and low-dose ibuprofen are associated with the lowest risk of CV events. COX-2 inhibitors cause fewer GI side effects than non-selective NSAIDs, but are associated with an increased risk of CV events. All NSAIDs including COX-2 inhibitors can cause renal impairment. Other adverse effects include **hypersensitivity reactions,** e.g. bronchospasm and angioedema, and **fluid retention,** which can worsen hypertension and heart failure.
Warnings	Avoid NSAIDs in ✖**severe renal impairment,** ✖**heart failure,** ✖**liver failure** and known ✖**NSAID hypersensitivity.** If NSAID use is unavoidable in patients at high risk of adverse effects (e.g. prior ▲**peptic ulcer disease** or ▲**GI bleeding,** ▲**cardiovascular disease,** ▲**renal impairment**), use the safest NSAID at the lowest effective dose for the shortest possible time.
Important interactions	Many drugs increase the risk of NSAID-related adverse effects including: *GI ulceration*: low-dose <u>aspirin</u>, <u>corticosteroids</u>; *GI bleeding*: anticoagulants, <u>SSRIs</u>, <u>venlafaxine</u>; *renal impairment:* <u>ACE inhibitors</u>, <u>diuretics</u>. NSAIDs increase the risk of bleeding with <u>warfarin</u> and reduce the therapeutic effects of antihypertensives and diuretics.

PRACTICAL PRESCRIBING

Prescription	NSAIDs are generally taken orally, but are also available as topical gels, suppositories and injectable preparations. Most NSAIDs have similar anti-inflammatory efficacy, but there may be considerable differences in individual patient response to and tolerance of individual drugs. The choice of drug and dosage will depend on the condition to be treated, as well as on safety considerations and patient choice. For example, in a patient with **rheumatoid arthritis,** naproxen 500 mg orally 12-hrly may be prescribed. Regular treatment for at least 3 weeks is required before full anti-inflammatory effect is seen, when treatment may be continued or switched to an alternative NSAID if ineffective. By contrast, a patient with **acute pain** may be treated with naproxen 250 mg orally 6–8-hrly as needed, to be stopped as soon as pain has resolved.
Administration	Oral NSAIDs should be taken with food to minimise GI upset.
Communication	Explain you are recommending an anti-inflammatory drug to help improve symptoms of pain, swelling and/or fever. Warn patients that the most common side effect is indigestion and advise them to stop treatment and seek medical advice if this occurs. For patients with acute pain, explain that long-term use, e.g. beyond 10 days, is not recommended due to the risk of side effects. Advise patients requiring long-term treatment (particularly if they have renal impairment) to stop NSAIDs if they become acutely unwell or dehydrated to reduce the risk of damage to the kidneys.
Monitoring	Control of pain and inflammation can be assessed by enquiry about symptoms, examination and by using scoring systems, e.g. a visual analogue scale for pain. Routine biochemical monitoring is not usually required but renal function should be monitored closely in patients with existing renal impairment. The NSAID should be stopped if there is significant deterioration.
Cost	NSAIDs are available in non-proprietary formulations, which are inexpensive. For patients who pay for their prescriptions, it may be cheaper for them to buy non-proprietary NSAIDs over the counter.

Clinical tip—Gastroprotection should be considered for all patients prescribed NSAIDs who are at increased risk of gastrointestinal complications. Risk factors include age >65 years, previous peptic ulcer disease, comorbidities (such as cardiovascular disease, diabetes), and concurrent therapy with other drugs with gastrointestinal side effects, particularly low-dose aspirin and prednisolone. The preferred strategy is to use ibuprofen with a proton pump inhibitor (e.g. lansoprazole 15 mg daily). Although COX-2 inhibitors are an alternative to this, they confer a higher risk of cardiovascular events.

Ocular lubricants (artificial tears)

CLINICAL PHARMACOLOGY

Common indications	❶ For first-line symptomatic treatment of **dry eye conditions** including **keratoconjunctivitis sicca** and **Sjögren's syndrome,** alongside environmental coping strategies and avoiding precipitants.
Mechanisms of action	In dry eye conditions, ocular lubricants have a **soothing effect** and help **protect the eye surfaces from abrasive damage.** Lubricant eye drops typically consist of an electrolyte solution with a viscosity agent, such as a cellulose polymer (e.g. hypromellose). Gels, such as carbomer 980 (the active ingredient of Viscotears®), have greater viscosity and are retained in the eye for longer. Ointments such as white soft paraffin with liquid paraffin (e.g. Lacri-Lube®) are highly viscous and may provide greater protection, but at a cost of causing blurred vision.
Important adverse effects	Ocular lubricants have **few side effects** other than mild **stinging** on application and temporary **blurring of vision.** The risk of blurring increases with viscosity and is therefore greatest for ointments. Unless specified as 'preservative-free,' it can be assumed that the preparation contains some form of preservative. This may incite a local **inflammatory (allergic) reaction** in some patients.
Warnings	As ocular lubricants are not absorbed, there are no major safety considerations from a systemic illness perspective.
Important interactions	There are no clinically important interactions.

hypromellose, carbomers, liquid and white soft paraffin

PRACTICAL PRESCRIBING

Prescription	Most ocular lubricants can be purchased from pharmacies without a prescription. In the absence of an underlying condition requiring medical supervision (such as Sjögren's syndrome), it is generally easier for the patient to purchase the product over the counter. Hypromellose 0.3% eye drops are usually tried first at a dose of 1–2 drops three times daily as required. They can be taken more often (up to hourly) if necessary, but if they are required more than four times daily on a regular basis, it may be worth trying a gel (e.g. Viscotears® 1 drop three times daily as required). In severe cases an ointment (e.g. Lacri-Lube®) may be added, although this is generally restricted to bedtime use due to its visual blurring effect.
Administration	Ocular lubricants are usually self-administered. After washing their hands, the patient tips their head back ('look at the ceiling') and pulls down slightly on their lower eyelid. Then, with the bottle held upside-down just above the eye, they squeeze to release a drop. For drops, they should then close their eye and press gently on the corner nearest the nose for 1 minute. For gels they should blink a few times to spread it over the eye. They should try not to let the tip of the dispenser touch their eye (or anything else), and should replace the cap directly after use to prevent infection.
Communication	Explain that you are recommending 'artificial tears' in the hope of improving their dry eyes. Explain how to take them and warn that, like most eye drops, they can sting a little when applied. This wears away quickly and they should then experience some relief from their dry eye symptoms. With continued use over days and weeks their symptoms may improve further as previous abrasive damage is repaired. They will probably need to take the treatment indefinitely.
Monitoring	The best form of monitoring is by the patient themselves. Ask them to return if their symptoms fail to improve or any problems develop.
Cost	Patients who pay for their prescription will generally save money if they purchase the product over the counter.

Clinical tip—If patients need to take more than one type of eye drop, the order of administration generally does not matter provided they are separated by at least 5 minutes (by which time most pharmacologically active agents will have been absorbed). The exception is ocular lubricants, which should be taken last so as to avoid being 'washed away' by the other eye drops.

Oestrogens and progestogens

CLINICAL PHARMACOLOGY

Common indications	❶ For **hormonal contraception** in women who require highly effective and reversible contraception, particularly if they may also benefit from its other effects, such as improved acne symptoms with oestrogens. ❷ For **hormone replacement therapy (HRT)** in women with **early menopause** (when it is given until 50 years of age) and those who have distressing **menopausal symptoms.**
Mechanisms of action	Luteinising hormone (LH) and follicle-stimulating hormone (FSH) control ovulation and ovarian production of oestrogen and progesterone. In turn, oestrogen and progesterone exert predominantly negative feedback on LH and FSH release. In hormonal contraception, an oestrogen (e.g. ethinylestradiol) and/or a progestogen (e.g. desogestrel) are given to **suppress LH/FSH release and hence ovulation.** Oestrogens and progestogens also have many effects outside the ovary. Some, such as those on the cervix and endometrium, may contribute to their contraceptive effect (this is especially important in progestogen-only contraception). Others offer additional benefits, e.g. reduced menstrual pain and bleeding, and improvements in acne. At the menopause, a fall in oestrogen and progesterone levels may generate a variety of symptoms, including vaginal dryness and vasomotor instability ('hot flushes'). Oestrogen replacement (usually with a progestogen) alleviates these.
Important adverse effects	Hormonal contraception may cause **irregular bleeding** and **mood changes.** It does not appear to cause weight gain. The oestrogens in combined hormonal contraception (CHC) products double the risk of **venous thromboembolism** (VTE), but the absolute risk is low. They also increase the risk of **cardiovascular disease** and **stroke,** but this is probably relevant only in women with other risk factors. They may be associated with increased risk of **breast and cervical cancer.** In both cases the effect is small, and for breast cancer, it gradually resolves after stopping the pill. Used alone (in progestogen-only pills), progestogens do not increase the risk of VTE or cardiovascular disease. The adverse effects of **hormone replacement therapy** are similar to those of CHC but, as the baseline rates are higher, the relative risks have more significant implications.
Warnings	All forms of oestrogens and progestogens are contraindicated in patients with ✗**breast cancer.** Combined hormonal contraception should be avoided in patients at increased risk for ▲**VTE** (past VTE; known thrombogenic mutation) or ▲**cardiovascular disease** (age >35 years; cardiovascular risk factors; migraine with aura; heavy smoking history).
Important interactions	Concurrent use of ▲**cytochrome P450 inducers** (e.g. rifampicin) may reduce the efficacy of hormonal contraception, particularly progestogen-only forms. Most other antibiotics are safe to use with hormonal contraception.

combined ethinylestradiol products, desogestrel

PRACTICAL PRESCRIBING

Prescription	Ideally, hormonal contraception should be prescribed only by appropriately-trained health professionals. CHC is commonly taken as a combined oral contraceptive (COC) pill. A preparation containing ethinylestradiol 30 or 35 micrograms is appropriate for most women. In patients with pre-existing medical conditions, the **UK Medical Eligibility Criteria for Contraceptive Use** from the Faculty of Sexual and Reproductive Healthcare provide a guide for prescribing. Often, where combined hormonal contraception is inappropriate, a progesterone-only pill may be suitable. For HRT, combined oestrogen–progestogen therapy is preferred, although women who have had a hysterectomy may receive oestrogen alone. For women with vaginal symptoms only, a vaginal oestrogen preparation is best.
Administration	COC pills can be started on any day of the cycle. If this is within the first 6 days, no additional contraception is needed. If it is beyond day 6, a barrier method should be used or sex avoided for the first 7 days. Most combined pills are designed to be taken for 21 days followed by a 7-day pill-free interval, during which a withdrawal bleed occurs. Some ('everyday') pills are taken throughout the cycle, but the tablets for days 22–28 are inactive. Guidance is available for **how to deal with missed pills;** this is summarised in the BNF. In general, missing 1 COC pill is okay, but missing 2 or more pills necessitates the use of additional contraception for the next 7 days.
Communication	Hormonal contraception should be offered only after a discussion of the risks and benefits of the various contraceptive methods available. Explain that the usual method of taking the pill (with either no pills or inactive pills in days 22–28) results in a bleed (not a 'period') each month, although irregular bleeding may occur initially. Explain the 'rules' for missed pills and provide written information to support this.
Monitoring	Baseline assessment should include a relevant history, blood pressure (BP) check and body mass index (BMI). A woman starting combined oral contraception should be seen again at 3 months to check her BP and to discuss any issues. Thereafter, she should be seen yearly to discuss health changes and to check her BP and BMI.
Cost	Hormonal contraception accounts for significant health expenditure. You should generally follow local policies on which pill to use. These take cost into account.

Clinical tip—Continuous or extended use of the combined oral contraceptive pill (without pill-free intervals) is unlicensed for most brands, but is safe and effective. It eliminates or reduces withdrawal bleeding, which some women may consider desirable.

Opioids, compound preparations

CLINICAL PHARMACOLOGY

Common indications	❶ **Mild-to-moderate pain:** as second-line agents when simple analgesics, such as <u>paracetamol</u>, are insufficient. Co-codamol and co-dydramol are on the second 'rung' of the World Health Organization (WHO) 'pain ladder'.
Mechanisms of action	The mechanism of action of <u>paracetamol</u> is poorly understood. Paracetamol is a **weak inhibitor of cyclooxygenase** (COX), the enzyme involved in prostaglandin metabolism. In the central nervous system, COX inhibition appears to increase the pain threshold. Codeine and dihydrocodeine are <u>weak opioids</u>. They are metabolised by cytochrome P450 enzymes to morphine and morphine-related metabolites. These metabolites, which are **agonists of opioid μ-receptors,** probably account for most of their analgesic effect (see <u>Opioids, strong</u>). Combining two analgesics with different mechanisms of action may offer better pain control than can be achieved with either drug alone. Putting them together in a fixed-ratio compound product improves convenience for the patient, although at a cost of reduced flexibility in terms of dose titration.
Important adverse effects	When taken at recommended doses, adverse effects from <u>paracetamol</u> are rare. Common side effects of codeine and dihydrocodeine include **nausea, constipation** and **drowsiness.** In overdose the effects of both paracetamol (principally hepatotoxocity) and opioid toxicity (neurological and respiratory depression) may be evident.
Warnings	Caution must be exercised when prescribing an opioid in the context of ▲**significant respiratory disease.** Codeine and dihydrocodeine rely on both the liver and the kidneys for their elimination. Doses should therefore be reduced in ▲**renal impairment** and ▲**hepatic impairment,** and also in the ▲**elderly.**
Important interactions	Opioids should ideally not be used with ▲**other sedating drugs** (e.g. <u>antipsychotics</u>, <u>benzodiazepines</u> and <u>tricyclic antidepressants</u>). Where their combination is unavoidable, closer monitoring is necessary.

co-codamol, co-dydramol

PRACTICAL PRESCRIBING

Prescription	Co-codamol and co-dydramol are only available as oral preparations. All tablets contain 500 mg of paracetamol, whereas the dose of the opioid varies. It is specified in the form 'co-codamol 8/500' or 'co-dydramol 10/500,' where the first number indicates the amount of opioid contained in each tablet (8 mg of codeine and 10 mg of dihydrocodeine in these examples, respectively). In mild–moderate chronic pain that has not responded to paracetamol you might, for example, change the paracetamol regimen to co-codamol 15/500, two tablets 6-hrly. This is effectively the same as adding codeine 30 mg 6-hrly to the existing paracetamol regimen, but with fewer pills (see Clinical tip). Whenever you prescribe an opioid for regular administration, you should consider prescribing a laxative. A <u>stimulant laxative</u> such as senna is a reasonable choice.
Administration	Doses should be taken at regular intervals with or without food.
Communication	Explain that you are offering a painkiller that is like a weaker version of morphine. It will work best if taken regularly at equal intervals. Discuss common side effects and, if appropriate, offer a laxative to prevent constipation. Advise patients to avoid driving or operating heavy machinery if they become drowsy or confused while taking the new painkiller. Mention that painkillers should always be stored out of reach of children. Advise patients not to take other medications that also contain paracetamol to avoid accidental overdose.
Monitoring	**Efficacy** of analgesics in pain control can be established by enquiry about symptoms or by using a pain score, e.g. a visual analogue scale. For mild-to-moderate acute pain, review the response to analgesia 1–2 hours after an oral dose. For chronic pain, schedule a review after 1–2 weeks to assess the need to step up or down the analgesic ladder, to assess **side effects,** and to consider the need for specialist referral.
Cost	Compound analgesics are available as inexpensive non-proprietary preparations. Branded preparations are more expensive. For patients who pay for prescriptions it may be cheaper to buy them over the counter.

Clinical tip—Compound analgesics offer some advantages in terms of convenience, and perhaps adherence. However, it is often preferable to use the drugs as separate products, at least initially. For example, you might prescribe codeine 15 mg tablets to be added to the patient's existing regimen of paracetamol 1 g 6-hrly. Under your guidance, the patient may then adjust the dose in the range 15–60 mg 6-hrly without having to obtain a new prescription each time. Having found the optimum balance between efficacy and side effects, it may *then* be appropriate to switch to the equivalent compound preparation.

Opioids, strong

CLINICAL PHARMACOLOGY

Common indications	❶ For rapid relief of **acute severe pain,** including post-operative pain and pain associated with acute myocardial infarction. ❷ For relief of **chronic pain,** when paracetamol, NSAIDs and weak opioids are insufficient ('rung 3' of the WHO pain ladder). ❸ For relief of **breathlessness** in the context of end-of-life care. ❹ To relieve breathlessness and anxiety in **acute pulmonary oedema,** alongside oxygen, furosemide and nitrates.
Mechanisms of action	The term *opioids* encompasses naturally-occurring *opiates* (e.g. morphine) plus *synthetic analogues* (e.g. oxycodone). Morphine and oxycodone are *strong opioids*. The therapeutic action of opioids arises from **activation of opioid μ (mu) receptors** in the central nervous system. Activation of these G protein-coupled receptors has several effects that, overall, reduce neuronal excitability and pain transmission. In the medulla, they blunt the response to hypoxia and hypercapnoea, reducing respiratory drive and breathlessness. By relieving pain, breathlessness and associated anxiety, opioids **reduce sympathetic nervous system (fight or flight) activity.** Thus, in myocardial infarction and acute pulmonary oedema they may reduce cardiac work and oxygen demand, as well as relieving symptoms. That said, although commonly used, the efficacy and safety of morphine in acute pulmonary oedema is not firmly established.
Important adverse effects	Opioids cause **respiratory depression** by reducing respiratory drive. They may cause euphoria and detachment, and in higher doses, **neurological depression.** They can activate the chemoreceptor trigger zone, causing **nausea and vomiting,** although this tends to settle with continued use. **Pupillary constriction** occurs due to stimulation of the Edinger–Westphal nucleus. In the large intestine, activation of μ receptors increases smooth muscle tone and reduces motility leading to **constipation.** In the skin, opioids may cause histamine release, leading to **itching,** urticaria, vasodilatation and sweating. Continued use can lead to **tolerance** (a state in which the dose required to produce the same effect increases over time) and **dependence.** Dependence becomes apparent on cessation of the opioid, when a **withdrawal reaction** occurs (see Clinical tip).
Warnings	Most opioids rely on the liver and the kidneys for elimination, so doses should be reduced in ▲hepatic failure and ▲renal impairment and in the ▲elderly. Do not give opioids in ▲respiratory failure except under senior guidance (e.g. in palliative care). Avoid opioids in ▲biliary colic, as they may cause spasm of the sphincter of Oddi, which may worsen pain.
Important interactions	Opioids should ideally not be used with ▲other sedating drugs (e.g. antipsychotics, benzodiazepines and tricyclic antidepressants). Where their combination is unavoidable, close monitoring is necessary.

PRACTICAL PRESCRIBING

Prescription	When treating **acute severe pain** in high dependency areas, morphine is given IV for rapid effect (onset at about 5 minutes). An initial dose of 2–10 mg, tailored to pain, age and other individual factors is prescribed in the once-only section. On a general ward, IM or SC administration is preferred. For **chronic pain,** the oral route is safest and usually most appropriate. Immediate-release oral morphine is preferred initially (e.g. Oramorph® 5 mg orally every 4 hours). Then, having found the optimum dose, this is converted to a modified-release form (e.g. MST Continus® 15 mg every 12 hours). Alongside regular treatment, 'breakthrough analgesia' should be prescribed. Prescribe immediate-release morphine at a dose of about one-sixth of the total daily regular dose (e.g. Oramorph® 5 mg 2-hrly) in the as-required section. For safety reasons, we favour **brand name prescribing** for strong oral opioids.
Administration	IV morphine should be given only in high dependency areas as adverse effects may be more pronounced. It should be given incrementally (1–2 mg every few minutes) to achieve the desired response.
Communication	Patients may be reluctant to accept morphine, due to the stigma associated with abuse and dependence. Explain that it is a highly effective painkiller and that 'addiction' is not an issue when it is used for pain control. That said, you should warn patients that the dose may need to be increased over time as they become tolerant to its effects; this is normal and should not cause alarm. Explain how the patient should take their morphine: e.g. to take 'slow-release' tablets every 12 hours for background pain and use 'fast-acting' solution when required for breakthrough pain. Explain that nausea usually settles after a few days, but offer an antiemetic (e.g. <u>metoclopramide</u>). Constipation is very common; pre-emptive use of a laxative (e.g. <u>senna</u>), along with good hydration, is advisable. Advise patients not to drive or operate heavy machinery if they feel drowsy or confused.
Monitoring	For **acute pain,** review your patients' response to analgesia within an hour, as well as for adverse effects such as respiratory depression. For **chronic pain,** schedule a review after a couple of weeks to assess the need to step up or down the analgesic ladder and/or specialist referral.
Cost	Morphine is relatively inexpensive. Synthetic opioids may be more expensive.

Clinical tip—The features of opioid withdrawal are the opposite of the clinical effects of opioids: anxiety, pain and breathlessness increase; the pupils dilate; and the skin is cool and dry with piloerection ('cold turkey'). Opioid dependence is less problematic when they are taken therapeutically rather than recreationally; do not let this concern deter you from offering opioids for severe or chronic pain, especially in end-of-life care.

Opioids, weak

CLINICAL PHARMACOLOGY

Common indications	❶ For **mild-to-moderate pain,** including post-operative pain, as second-line agents when simple analgesics, such as <u>paracetamol</u>, are insufficient. Weak opioids are on the second rung of the World Health Organization pain ladder.
Mechanisms of action	In unmodified form, codeine and dihydrocodeine are very weak opioids. They are metabolised in the liver to produce relatively small amounts of morphine (from codeine) or dihydromorphine (from dihydrocodeine). These metabolites, which are stronger **agonists of opioid μ (mu) receptors** (see <u>Opioids, strong</u>), probably account for most of the analgesic effect. About 10% of Caucasians have a less active form of the key metabolising enzyme (called cytochrome P450 2D6), and these people may find codeine and dihydrocodine largely ineffective. Tramadol is a synthetic analogue of codeine; it is perhaps best classified as a 'moderate' strength opioid. Like codeine, tramadol and its active metabolite are μ-receptor agonists. Unlike other opioids, tramadol also affects serotonergic and adrenergic pathways, where it is thought to act as a serotonin and noradrenaline reuptake inhibitor. This probably contributes to its analgesic effect.
Important adverse effects	Common side effects of weak opioids include **nausea, constipation, dizziness** and **drowsiness.** All opioids can cause **neurological and respiratory depression** when taken in overdose. Tramadol may cause less constipation and respiratory depression than other opioids. **Codeine and dihydrocodeine must never be given intravenously,** as this can cause a severe reaction similar to anaphylaxis. This is mediated by histamine release, but does not have an 'allergic' basis.
Warnings	Caution must be exercised when prescribing an opioid in the context of ▲**significant respiratory disease.** Tramadol, codeine and dihydrocodeine rely on both the liver and the kidneys for their elimination. Doses should therefore be reduced in ▲**renal impairment** and ▲**hepatic impairment,** and also in the ▲**elderly.** Tramadol lowers the seizure threshold so is best avoided in patients with ▲**epilepsy,** and certainly should not be used in those with ✖**uncontrolled epilepsy.**
Important interactions	Opioids should ideally not be used with ▲**other sedating drugs** (e.g. <u>antipsychotics</u>, <u>benzodiazepines</u> and <u>tricyclic antidepressants</u>). Where their combination is unavoidable, closer monitoring is necessary. Tramadol should not be used with other ▲**drugs that lower the seizure threshold,** such as <u>serotonin-selective reuptake inhibitors</u> and <u>tricyclic antidepressants.</u>

tramadol, codeine, dihydrocodeine

PRACTICAL PRESCRIBING

Prescription	Opioids should be prescribed orally wherever possible. Preparations are available for IM injection, but their use is largely restricted to the operating theatre. Regular prescription is usually preferable to as-required prescription to avoid the need for 'catch-up' analgesia. A common starting prescription might be for codeine or dihydrocodeine 30 mg orally 4-hrly, or tramadol 50 mg orally 4-hrly. Whenever you prescribe an opioid for regular administration you should consider prescribing a laxative. A <u>stimulant laxative</u> such as senna is a reasonable choice.
Administration	Doses should be taken at regular intervals. They may be taken with or without food. If they are being administered intramuscularly, care must be taken to avoid inadvertent IV administration.
Communication	Explain that you are offering a painkiller that is like a weaker version of morphine. It will work best if taken regularly at equal intervals. Discuss common side effects, and if appropriate, offer a laxative to prevent constipation. Advise patients to avoid driving or operating heavy machinery if they become drowsy or confused while taking the new painkiller. Mention that painkillers should always be stored out of reach of children.
Monitoring	For mild-to-moderate acute pain, review the response to analgesia 1–2 hours after an oral dose. For chronic pain, schedule a review after 1–2 weeks to assess the need to step up or down the analgesic ladder, to assess side effects, and to consider the need for specialist referral.
Cost	Weak opioids are available in inexpensive non-proprietary forms. Avoid using expensive branded products, such as modified-release tramadol, unless there is a clear reason to do so.

Clinical tip—Anaesthetists may sometimes give an IM injection of codeine towards the end of an operation, while the patient is still under general anaesthesia, to provide post-operative analgesia. This may cause a red patch to form at the injection site (which, for reasons of accessibility, is usually the lateral aspect of the thigh). Patients and clinical staff may notice this and wonder what it is and whether it has any significance. It is mediated by histamine release and, provided it is not progressive, is no cause for alarm.

Oxygen

CLINICAL PHARMACOLOGY

Common indications	❶ To increase tissue oxygen delivery in states of **hypoxaemia.** ❷ To accelerate reabsorption of pleural gas in **pneumothorax.** ❸ To reduce the half-life of carboxyhaemoglobin in **carbon monoxide poisoning.**
Mechanisms of action	An abnormally low partial pressure of oxygen (PO_2) in arterial blood (PaO_2), termed hypoxaemia, may be a consequence of a wide range of disease processes. Its effect is to reduce the delivery of oxygen to tissues (hypoxia), forcing them to use anaerobic metabolism for energy generation. Supplemental oxygen therapy increases the PO_2 in alveolar gas, driving more rapid diffusion of oxygen into blood. The resultant increase in PaO_2 **increases delivery of oxygen to the tissues,** which in effect 'buys time' while the underlying disease is corrected. In *pneumothorax,* supplemental oxygen therapy has an additional benefit of reducing the fraction of nitrogen in alveolar gas. This **accelerates the diffusion of nitrogen out of the body.** Since pleural air is composed mostly of nitrogen, this increases its rate of reabsorption. In *carbon monoxide (CO) poisoning,* oxygen competes with CO to bind with haemoglobin and thereby **shortens the half-life of carboxyhaemoglobin,** returning haemoglobin to a form that can again transport oxygen to tissues.
Important adverse effects	The most common adverse effects of oxygen are related to the delivery device (e.g. the **discomfort of a facemask**) or its lack of water vapour (**dry throat**). The latter can be improved by using a humidification system. Except in pneumothorax and carbon monoxide poisoning, there is little to be gained from an *abnormally high* PaO_2 and, indeed, there is some evidence that this may be harmful. However, this concern should not lead you to withhold oxygen in critical illness or states of severe hypoxaemia, in which oxygen may be life-saving.
Warnings	Patients with ▲**chronic type 2 respiratory failure** (e.g. those with severe COPD) exhibit a number of adaptive changes in response to persistent hypoxaemia and hypercapnoea. If exposed to high inspired oxygen concentrations, this finely balanced adaptive state may be disturbed, resulting in a rise in the blood carbon dioxide concentration. This may lead to respiratory acidosis, depressed consciousness, and worsened tissue hypoxia. This necessitates a different approach to oxygen therapy (see Prescription and Administration). Oxygen accelerates combustion and therefore presents a fire risk if it is brought into close proximity with a ✖**heat source or naked flame,** including from smoking.
Important interactions	There are no clinically important interactions.

PRACTICAL PRESCRIBING

Prescription	Oxygen therapy should always be guided by a written prescription, except in emergencies when it may initially be administered without a prescription. The oxygen prescription is usually found on a dedicated section of the drug chart or a separate chart. Its key feature is the **target oxygen saturation range,** as measured by pulse oximetry (SpO₂). The target SpO₂ should be 94–98% in most patients and 88–92% in those with chronic type 2 respiratory failure. For the **initial delivery device,** in general, prescribe a reservoir mask in critical illness and patients with SpO₂ <85%; a Venturi mask (28%) for patients in chronic type 2 respiratory failure; and nasal cannulae for everyone else.
Administration	**Reservoir (non-rebreathing) masks** have a bag (reservoir) that is continuously filled by the incoming oxygen supply. Inspired gas is drawn from the bag so contains a high oxygen concentration (at least 60–80%). The oxygen flow rate should be 15 L/min. **Venturi masks** blend oxygen with air in a fixed ratio. The oxygen concentration is defined by the characteristics of the device. It is identified by a colour coding system and written information on the device. This will also specify the oxygen flow rate that, when entrained air is taken into account, produces a total gas flow rate sufficient to maintain a fixed inspired oxygen concentration. **Nasal cannulae** deliver a variable oxygen concentration (roughly 24–50% at flow rates of 2–6 L/min). **Simple facemasks** are also variable performance devices; they have few advantages over nasal cannulae and are less comfortable.
Communication	Explain that the facemask or nasal cannulae should generally be kept in place continuously, but may briefly be removed to allow eating and drinking. Ask them to report any discomfort, as it may be possible to improve this with a different device or the addition of humidification.
Monitoring	**Frequent SpO₂ monitoring** is essential in all patients receiving oxygen for acute illness. The device and/or flow rate should be adjusted as necessary to keep the SpO₂ within the target range. In addition, **arterial blood gas measurement** is essential in patients with critical illness; those with chronic type 2 respiratory failure or at risk of hypercapnoea; and those with hypoxaemia that is unexpected, progressive, or disproportionate to their illness.
Cost	The cost of oxygen is not material to decisions regarding its use.

Clinical tip—Remember that the PaO_2 is only one determinant of the amount of oxygen reaching the tissues. Equally important are the haemoglobin concentration and the cardiac output. Neglecting to correct these, if they are significantly abnormal, may render oxygen therapy worthless.

Paracetamol

CLINICAL PHARMACOLOGY

Common indications	❶ Paracetamol is a first-line analgesic for most forms of **acute and chronic pain.** The WHO pain ladder (originally designed to guide the treatment of cancer pain) uses regular paracetamol as the basis of treatment, with <u>weak</u> then <u>strong opioids</u> added incrementally until pain is controlled. ❷ Paracetamol is an antipyretic that can reduce **fever** and its associated symptoms (e.g. shivering).
Mechanisms of action	The mechanisms of action of paracetamol are **poorly understood.** Paracetamol is a **weak inhibitor of cyclooxygenase** (COX), the enzyme involved in prostaglandin metabolism. In the central nervous system, COX inhibition appears to increase the pain threshold and reduce prostaglandin (PGE_2) concentrations in the thermoregulatory region of the hypothalamus, controlling fever. Paracetamol has specificity for COX-2 (the isoform induced in inflammation) rather than COX-1 (the isoform involved in protecting the gastric mucosa and regulating renal blood flow and clotting). However, despite its COX-2 selectivity, paracetamol is a weak anti-inflammatory, as its actions are inhibited in inflammatory lesions by the presence of peroxides.
Important adverse effects	At treatment doses, paracetamol is very safe with **few side effects.** Lack of COX-1 inhibition means that it does not cause peptic ulceration or renal impairment or precipitate cardiovascular events (unlike <u>NSAIDs</u>). Its safety makes it a popular choice as a first-line analgesic. In **overdose,** paracetamol causes **liver failure.** Paracetamol is metabolised by cytochrome P450 enzymes to a toxic metabolite (N-acetyl-p-benzoquinone imine [NAPQI]), which is conjugated with glutathione before elimination. After overdose, this elimination pathway is saturated, and NAPQI accumulation causes hepatocellular necrosis. Hepatotoxicity can be prevented by treatment with the glutathione precursor <u>acetylcysteine</u>.
Warnings	Paracetamol dose should be reduced in people at increased risk of liver toxicity, either because of *increased NAPQI production* (e.g. in ▲**chronic excessive alcohol use,** inducing metabolising enzymes) or *reduced glutathione stores* (e.g. in ▲**malnutrition,** ▲**low body weight** (<50 kg) and ▲**severe hepatic impairment**). This is particularly important where paracetamol is given by IV infusion.
Important interactions	There are few clinically significant interactions between paracetamol and other drugs. **Cytochrome P450 inducers**, e.g. <u>phenytoin</u> and <u>carbamazepine,</u> increase the rate of NAPQI production and risk of liver toxicity **after paracetamol overdose.**

paracetamol

PRACTICAL PRESCRIBING

Prescription	**Oral paracetamol** is on the 'general sales list', which means that it can be purchased from any retail outlet, although it is also available on prescription. For patients unable to take drugs by mouth, paracetamol can be prescribed for **IV infusion** or **rectal** administration. By all routes, the **usual adult dose** is 0.5–1 g every 4–6 hours, maximum 4 g daily (see Warnings). Paracetamol can be prescribed for **regular** administration or to be taken only **as required,** depending on the nature of the pain. When prescribed 'as required' the maximum daily dose must always be stated.
Administration	**Oral paracetamol** is available as tablets, caplets, capsules, soluble tablets and oral suspension. **Intravenous paracetamol** is pre-prepared as a solution that can be infused undiluted over 15 minutes or diluted in 0.9% sodium chloride or 5% glucose solution before administration.
Communication	Explain that you are prescribing paracetamol with the aim of reducing or relieving pain. Effects should be felt around half an hour after taking it. Where regular paracetamol is prescribed, explain the importance of taking it every 6 hours. Warn them not to exceed the recommended **maximum daily dose** because of the potential risk of liver poisoning. Advise them that many medicines purchased from the chemist (e.g. **cold and flu preparations**) contain paracetamol. Warn them to check the label or ask the pharmacist before taking these with paracetamol.
Monitoring	**Efficacy** of paracetamol in pain control can be established by enquiry about symptoms or by using a pain score, e.g. a visual analogue scale. For acute pain, review response to analgesia 1–2 hours after an oral dose. For chronic pain, schedule a review to assess the need to step up or down the analgesic ladder. After **overdose,** blood tests including international normalised ratio (INR), serum alanine aminotransferase (ALT) activity and creatinine concentration are required to establish efficacy of acetylcysteine treatment and determine the need for further treatment.
Cost	A single dose of **oral paracetamol** 1 g can cost as little as 2p. Advise patients purchasing paracetamol from a shop or pharmacist to ask for the cheapest brand. As **IV paracetamol** is around 60 times more expensive (£1.25 for 1 g plus infusion costs) than oral formulations, it should be reserved for patients unable to take medicines by mouth and administration should be switched from IV to oral as soon as possible.

Clinical tip—If you are writing up paracetamol on an inpatient chart, always check that it has not already been prescribed. For example, if you are prescribing paracetamol regularly, cross it off the 'as required' side. Look out for 'co-' drugs such as co-codamol or co-dydramol with 'hidden' paracetamol.

Penicillins

CLINICAL PHARMACOLOGY

Common indications	❶ Streptococcal infection, including **tonsillitis, pneumonia** (in combination with a <u>macrolide</u> if severe), **endocarditis** and **skin and soft tissue infections** (added to <u>flucloxacillin</u> if severe). ❷ Clostridial infection, for example **tetanus.** ❸ Meningococcal infection, for example **meningitis, septicaemia.**
Mechanisms of action	Penicillins inhibit the enzymes responsible for cross-linking peptidoglycans in bacterial cell walls. This **weakens cell walls,** preventing them from maintaining an osmotic gradient. Uncontrolled entry of water into bacteria causes **cell swelling, lysis and death.** Penicillins contain a β-**lactam ring,** which is responsible for their antimicrobial activity. **Side chains** attached to the β-lactam ring can be modified to make semi-synthetic penicillins. The nature of the side chain determines the antimicrobial spectrum and other properties of the drug. Bacteria **resist** the actions of penicillins by making β-**lactamase,** an enzyme which breaks the β-lactam ring and prevents antimicrobial activity. Other mechanisms of resistance include limiting the intracellular concentration of penicillin (reduced bacterial permeability or increased extrusion) or changes in the target enzyme to prevent penicillin binding.
Important adverse effects	Penicillin **allergy** affects 1–10% of people. This usually presents as a **skin rash** 7–10 days after first exposure or 1–2 days after repeat exposure (subacute [delayed] IgG-mediated reaction). Less commonly, an immediate (minutes to hours) life-threatening IgE-mediated **anaphylactic reaction** occurs with some or all of hypotension, bronchial and laryngeal spasm/oedema and angioedema. **Central nervous system toxicity** (including convulsions and coma) can occur with high doses of penicillin or where severe renal impairment delays excretion.
Warnings	Penicillin can generally be used safely in most clinical situations, although a dose reduction is required for patients with ▲**renal impairment.** The main contraindication to penicillin use is a ✖**history of penicillin allergy.** Note that allergy to one type of penicillin implies allergy to all types as it is due to a reaction to the basic penicillin structure.
Important interactions	Penicillins reduce renal excretion of ▲<u>methotrexate</u>, increasing the risk of toxicity.

benzylpenicillin, phenoxymethylpenicillin

PRACTICAL PRESCRIBING

Prescription	*Benzylpenicillin* can only be administered by injection (IV or IM), as hydrolysis by gastric acid prevents gastrointestinal absorption. It is prescribed for the treatment of severe infections, usually at a high dose (e.g. 1.2 g 4–6-hrly). *Phenoxymethylpenicillin* ('penicillin V') is stable in the presence of gastric acid so can be taken orally as tablets or in solution. As absorption is unpredictable and phenoxymethylpenicillin is less active than benzylpenicillin, it is not used for severe infections. Benzylpenicillin and phenoxymethylpenicillin have a short plasma half-life of 30–60 minutes due to rapid renal excretion so need to be administered 4–6-hrly. When writing an inpatient prescription for antibiotics, it is essential to include the indication and duration of treatment to promote review and ensure good antibiotic stewardship.
Administration	IV benzylpenicillin can be given either as a slow IV injection or by infusion.
Communication	Explain that the aim of treatment is to get rid of infection and improve symptoms. For oral treatment, encourage the patient to complete the prescribed course. Before prescribing, always check with your patient personally or get collateral history to ensure that they do not have an **allergy** to any form of penicillin or other β-lactam antibiotics. Warn them to seek medical advice if a rash or other unexpected symptoms develop. If an allergy develops during treatment, give the patient written and verbal advice not to take this antibiotic in the future and make sure that the reaction is clearly documented in their medical records.
Monitoring	Check that infection resolves by resolution of symptoms, signs (e.g. pyrexia, lung crackles) and blood markers (e.g. falling C-reactive protein and white cell count) as appropriate.
Cost	Both benzylpenicillin and phenoxymethylpenicillin are inexpensive. Cost is not a consideration when choosing between these preparations.

Clinical tip—Where antibiotics are required to treat a young person with a sore throat caused by an unknown organism, make sure you choose phenoxymethylpenicillin, not amoxicillin. If the sore throat is due to Epstein-Barr virus (glandular fever), amoxicillin treatment commonly causes a rash. Although this is not truly an allergic reaction, it may lead to a lifetime label of penicillin allergy for that patient.

Penicillins, antipseudomonal

CLINICAL PHARMACOLOGY

Common indications	Antipseudomonal penicillins are reserved for **severe infections,** particularly where there is a **broad spectrum of potential pathogens** (including *Pseudomonas aeruginosa*); **antibiotic resistance** is likely (e.g. hospital-acquired infection); or patients are **immunocompromised** (e.g. neutropenia). Clinical infections treated with these drugs include: ❶ Lower respiratory tract infection. ❷ Urinary tract infection. ❸ Intra-abdominal sepsis. ❹ Skin and soft tissue infection.
Mechanisms of action	Penicillins inhibit the enzymes responsible for cross-linking peptidoglycans in bacterial cell walls. This **weakens cell walls,** preventing them from maintaining an osmotic gradient. Uncontrolled entry of water into bacteria causes **cell swelling, lysis and death.** Penicillins contain a **β-lactam ring,** which is responsible for their antimicrobial activity. **Side chains** attached to the β-lactam ring can be modified to make semi-synthetic penicillins. For piperacillin, the side chain of <u>broad-spectrum penicillins</u> has been converted to a form of urea. This longer side chain may improve affinity to penicillin binding proteins, increasing the spectrum of antimicrobial activity to include *Pseudomonas aeruginosa.* Addition of the β-lactamase inhibitor **tazobactam** confers antimicrobial **activity against β-lactamase-producing bacteria** (e.g. *Staphylococcus aureus*, Gram-negative anaerobes).
Important adverse effects	**Gastrointestinal upset** including nausea and diarrhoea is common. Less frequently, **antibiotic-associated colitis** occurs when broad-spectrum antibiotics kill normal gastrointestinal flora, allowing overgrowth of toxin-producing *Clostridium difficile*. This is debilitating and can be complicated by colonic perforation and/or death. Delayed or immediate **hypersensitivity** may occur (see <u>Penicillins</u>).
Warnings	Antipseudomonal penicillins should be used with caution in people ▲**at risk of *C. difficile* infection,** particularly those in hospital and the elderly. The main contraindication is a ✖**history of penicillin allergy.** Note that allergy to one type of penicillin implies allergy to all types as it is due to a reaction to the basic penicillin structure. The dose of antipseudomonal penicillins should be reduced in patients with ▲**moderate/severe renal impairment.**
Important interactions	Penicillins reduce renal excretion of ▲<u>methotrexate</u>, increasing the risk of toxicity. Antipseudomonal penicillins can enhance the anticoagulant effect of <u>warfarin</u> by killing normal gastrointestinal flora that synthesise vitamin K.

piperacillin with tazobactam (e.g. Tazocin®)

PRACTICAL PRESCRIBING

Prescription	Piperacillin is always given with tazobactam. It can be prescribed by non-proprietary name (piperacillin with tazobactam) or brand name (Tazocin®). Piperacillin with tazobactam can only be given by IV infusion. Thus, the whole course (usually 5–14 days) has to be given IV as no oral switch is possible. The usual dose is 4.5 g, containing 4 g of piperacillin and 500 mg of tazobactam, given every 6–8 hours. When writing an inpatient prescription for antibiotics, it is essential to include the indication and duration of treatment to promote review and ensure good antibiotic stewardship.
Administration	Piperacillin with tazobactam is formulated as a powder to be reconstituted in 10 mL sterile water or <u>0.9% sodium chloride</u>. This is diluted further in 50–150 mL of <u>0.9% sodium chloride</u> or <u>5% glucose</u> for IV infusion over 30 minutes.
Communication	Explain that the aim of treatment is to get rid of infection and improve symptoms. Before prescribing, always check with your patient personally or get collateral history to ensure that they do not have an **allergy** to any form of penicillin or other β-lactam antibiotics. Warn them to seek medical advice if a rash or other unexpected symptoms develop. If an allergy develops during treatment, give the patient written and verbal advice not to take this antibiotic in the future and make sure that the allergy is clearly documented in their medical records.
Monitoring	Check that infection resolves by resolution of symptoms, signs (e.g. pyrexia, lung crackles) and blood markers (e.g. falling C-reactive protein and white cell count) as appropriate.
Cost	Non-proprietary piperacillin with tazobactam is cheaper than branded Tazocin®. As this is a hospital-only drug, local pharmacy purchasing arrangements will determine which one is supplied irrespective of what you prescribe.

Clinical tip—Each dose of piperacillin with tazobactam contains about 10 mmol Na^+ and is infused in 50–150 mL fluid. Take this into account when determining the need for supplementary fluid, particularly in patients with heart failure.

Penicillins, broad-spectrum

CLINICAL PHARMACOLOGY

Common indications	❶ Empirical treatment of **pneumonia,** which may be caused by Gram-positive (e.g. *Streptococcus pneumoniae*) or Gram-negative pathogens (e.g. *Haemophilus influenzae*). ❷ Empirical treatment of **urinary tract infection** (most commonly caused by *Escherichia coli*). <u>Trimethoprim</u> and <u>nitrofurantoin</u> are alternatives. ❸ As part of combination treatment (as co-amoxiclav) for **hospital-acquired infection** or **intra-abdominal sepsis,** which may be caused by Gram-negative and anaerobic pathogens or antibiotic-resistant organisms. ❹ As part of combination treatment for ***H. pylori*-associated peptic ulcers.**
Mechanisms of action	Penicillins inhibit the enzymes responsible for cross-linking peptidoglycans in bacterial cell walls. This **weakens cell walls,** preventing them from maintaining an osmotic gradient. Uncontrolled entry of water into bacteria causes **cell swelling, lysis** and **death.** Penicillins contain a β-**lactam ring,** which is responsible for their antimicrobial activity. **Side chains** attached to the β-lactam ring can be modified to make semi-synthetic penicillins. For amoxicillin, addition of an amino group to the side chain increases activity against aerobic Gram-negative bacteria, making this a 'broad-spectrum' antibiotic. Addition of the β-lactamase inhibitor **clavulanic acid** (creating co-amoxiclav) increases the spectrum of antimicrobial activity further to include β-**lactamase-producing bacteria** (e.g. *Staphylococcus aureus*, Gram-negative anaerobes).
Important adverse effects	**Gastrointestinal upset** such as nausea and diarrhoea are common. Less frequently, **antibiotic-associated colitis** occurs when broad-spectrum antibiotics kill normal gut flora, allowing overgrowth of toxin-producing *Clostridium difficile.* This is debilitating and can be complicated by colonic perforation and/or death. Penicillin **allergy** affects 1–10% of people. This usually presents as a **skin rash** 7–10 days after first or 1–2 days after repeat exposure (delayed IgG-mediated reaction). Less commonly, an immediate (minutes to hours) life-threatening IgE-mediated **anaphylactic reaction** occurs with features including hypotension, bronchospasm and angiooedema. **Cholestatic jaundice** is a rare adverse effect of co-amoxiclav.
Warnings	Broad-spectrum penicillins should be used with caution in people ▲**at risk of *C. difficile* infection,** particularly those in hospital and the elderly. The main contraindication to the use of broad-spectrum penicillins is a ✖**history of penicillin allergy.** Note that allergy to one type of penicillin implies allergy to all types as it is due to a reaction to the basic penicillin structure. The dose of broad-spectrum penicillins should be reduced in patients with ✖**severe renal impairment** (risk of crystalluria).
Important interactions	Penicillins reduce renal excretion of ▲<u>methotrexate</u>, increasing the risk of toxicity. Broad-spectrum penicillins can enhance the anticoagulant effect of <u>warfarin</u> by killing normal gut flora that synthesise vitamin K.

PRACTICAL PRESCRIBING

Prescription	For **severe infection,** *amoxicillin* is prescribed at a high dose (e.g. 1 g 8-hrly) for IV administration. Intravenous antibiotics should be switched to oral administration after 48 hours if clinically indicated and the patient is improving (e.g. resolution of pyrexia, tachycardia) and able to take oral medication. **Prompt IV-to-oral switch** reduces complications and costs of antibiotic treatment and facilitates early discharge. For **mild-to-moderate infection** (e.g. without systemic features) oral amoxicillin should be prescribed at a lower dose (e.g. 250–500 mg 8-hrly). Where *co-amoxiclav* is prescribed, the strength (e.g. co-amoxiclav 500/125) indicates the relative amounts of amoxicillin (e.g. 500 mg) and clavulanic acid (e.g. 125 mg) in the preparation (in practice the dose prescribed is often these numbers combined, e.g. 625 mg). When writing an inpatient prescription for antibiotics, it is essential to include the **indication and duration of treatment** to promote review and ensure good antibiotic stewardship.
Communication	Explain that the aim of treatment is to get rid of infection and improve symptoms. For oral treatment, encourage the patient to complete the prescribed course. Before prescribing, always check with your patient personally or get collateral history to ensure that they do not have an **allergy** to any form of penicillin or other β-lactam antibiotics. Warn them to seek medical advice if a rash or other unexpected symptoms develop. If an allergy develops during treatment, give the patient written and verbal advice not to take this antibiotic in the future and make sure that the allergy is clearly documented in their medical records.
Monitoring	Check that infection resolves by resolution of symptoms, signs (e.g. pyrexia, lung crackles) and blood markers (e.g. falling C-reactive protein and white cell count) as appropriate.
Cost	When prescribing *co-amoxiclav*, always use this non-proprietary name rather than the brand name, allowing dispensing of the cheapest preparation. Following this simple rule could save the NHS around a quarter of a million pounds per year!

Clinical tip—Individual hospitals have antibiotic policies to reduce the risk of hospital-acquired infection. These include limiting the use of broad-spectrum antibiotics such as amoxicillin/co-amoxiclav where there is a narrower spectrum alternative. For example, they may recommend benzylpenicillin rather than amoxicillin for pneumonia alongside clarithromycin. Always get to know and follow your local antibiotic guidelines and seek microbiology advice where these do not cover a specific clinical situation.

Penicillins, penicillinase-resistant

CLINICAL PHARMACOLOGY

Common indications	Staphylococcal infection, including: ❶ **Skin and soft tissue infections** such as cellulitis (in combination with <u>benzylpenicillin</u> for more severe infection). ❷ **Osteomyelitis** and **septic arthritis.** ❸ Other infections, including **endocarditis.**

Mechanisms of action	Penicillins inhibit the enzymes responsible for cross-linking peptidoglycans in bacterial cell walls. This **weakens cell walls,** preventing them from maintaining an osmotic gradient. Uncontrolled entry of water into bacteria causes **cell swelling, lysis** and **death.**
	   Penicillins contain a **β-lactam ring,** which is responsible for their antimicrobial activity. **Side chains** attached to the β-lactam ring can be modified to make semi-synthetic penicillins. The nature of the side chain determines the antimicrobial spectrum and other properties of the drug.
	   For flucloxacillin, an acyl side chain protects the β-lactam ring from β-lactamases, which are enzymes made by bacteria to deactivate penicillin. This makes flucloxacillin **effective against β-lactamase producing staphylococci.** Meticillin-resistant *Staphylococcus aureus* (MRSA) resists the actions of flucloxacillin by reducing penicillin binding affinity.

Important adverse effects	Minor **gastrointestinal upset** is common. Penicillin **allergy** affects 1–10% of people. This usually presents as a **skin rash** 7–10 days after first exposure or 1–2 days after repeat exposure (delayed IgG-mediated reaction). Less commonly, an immediate (minutes to hours) life-threatening IgE-mediated **anaphylactic reaction** occurs with some or all of hypotension, bronchial and laryngeal spasm/oedema and angioedema. **Liver toxicity,** including cholestasis and hepatitis, is a rare but serious adverse effect which can occur even after treatment has been completed. **Central nervous system toxicity** (for example convulsions, coma) can occur with high doses of penicillin or where severe renal impairment delays excretion.
Warnings	Flucloxacillin can generally be used safely in most situations, although a dose reduction is required for patients with ▲**renal failure.** The main contraindication to flucloxacillin use is a ✖**history of penicillin allergy.** Note that allergy to one type of penicillin implies allergy to all types as it is due to a reaction to the basic penicillin structure. Flucloxacillin is also contraindicated in patients with ✖**prior flucloxacillin-related hepatotoxicity.**
Important interactions	Penicillins reduce renal excretion of ▲<u>methotrexate</u>, increasing the risk of toxicity.

PRACTICAL PRESCRIBING

Prescription	Flucloxacillin is prescribed at high dose (e.g. 1–2 g 6-hrly) for IV administration for severe infection (e.g. where patients are systemically unwell). A prolonged course (e.g. 6 weeks) of high-dose IV flucloxacillin may be required for deep-seated infections such as osteomyelitis or endocarditis. Patients with less severe infection (such as cellulitis without systemic illness) can be prescribed flucloxacillin orally at a lower dose, e.g. 250–500 mg. Flucloxacillin has a short plasma half-life of 45–60 minutes due to rapid renal excretion, so needs to be administered 6-hrly. When writing an inpatient prescription for antibiotics, it is essential to include the indication and duration of treatment to promote review and ensure good antibiotic stewardship.
Administration	IV flucloxacillin can be given either as a slow IV injection or by infusion. Oral flucloxacillin is available as capsules or as oral solutions (elixir or syrup) for infants and those with difficulty swallowing.
Communication	Explain that the aim of treatment is to get rid of infection and improve symptoms. For oral treatment, encourage the patient to complete the prescribed course. Before prescribing, always check with your patient personally or get collateral history to ensure that they do not have an **allergy** to any form of penicillin or other β-lactam antibiotics. Warn them to seek medical advice if a rash or other unexpected symptoms develop. If an allergy develops during treatment, give the patient written and verbal advice not to take this antibiotic in the future and make sure that the allergy is clearly documented in their medical records.
Monitoring	Check that infection resolves by resolution of symptoms, signs (e.g. pyrexia, erythema of cellulitis) and blood markers (e.g. falling C-reactive protein and white cell count) as appropriate.
Cost	Flucloxacillin is inexpensive in IV or oral forms.

Clinical tip—Many patients will say they are 'allergic' to penicillin. Check this is a true hypersensitivity, with features of skin rash, bronchospasm or anaphylaxis, rather than a dose-related side effect such as severe vomiting. A **✗prior anaphylactic reaction** to any penicillin is an **absolute contraindication** to prescription of any penicillin or other β-lactam antibiotic, whereas you can prescribe these antibiotics to intolerant patients (perhaps with an antiemetic) where there is a strong indication.

Phenytoin

CLINICAL PHARMACOLOGY

Common indications	❶ To control seizures in **status epilepticus** where benzodiazepines are ineffective. ❷ To reduce the frequency of generalised or focal seizures in **epilepsy**, although drugs with fewer adverse effects and interactions (e.g. valproate, lamotrigine, levetiracetam) are usually preferred.
Mechanisms of action	The mechanism of action of phenytoin is incompletely understood. Phenytoin **reduces neuronal excitability** and electrical conductance among brain cells, which inhibits the spread of seizure activity. It appears to do this by binding to **neuronal Na⁺ channels** in their inactive state, prolonging inactivity and preventing Na⁺ influx into the neuron. This prevents a drift in membrane potential from the resting (–70 mV) to the threshold (–55 mV) value required to trigger an action potential. A similar effect in **cardiac Purkinje fibres** may account for both antiarrhythmic and cardiotoxic effects of phenytoin.
Important adverse effects	Long-term phenytoin treatment can cause a **change in appearance,** with skin coarsening, acne, hirsutism and gum hypertrophy. Dose-related **neurological effects** include cerebellar toxicity (e.g. nystagmus, ataxia and discoordination) and impaired cognition or consciousness. Phenytoin can cause **haematological disorders** and **osteomalacia** by inducing folic acid and vitamin D metabolism. **Hypersensitivity** reactions to phenytoin range from mild skin rash to the rare life-threatening antiepileptic hypersensitivity syndrome (see Carbamazepine). Phenytoin toxicity (due to overdose or injudicious IV infusion) can cause death through **cardiovascular collapse** and **respiratory depression.**
Warnings	Phenytoin is metabolised by the liver with **zero-order kinetics** (i.e. at a constant rate irrespective of plasma concentrations) for concentrations at or above the therapeutic range. Moreover, the **therapeutic index is low,** implying that the safety margin between therapeutic and toxic doses is narrow. Phenytoin dosage should therefore be reduced in ▲**hepatic impairment**. *In utero* phenytoin exposure is associated with craniofacial abnormalities and reduced IQ (**fetal hydantoin syndrome**). Women with epilepsy planning ▲**pregnancy** should discuss treatment with a specialist and take high-dose folic acid before conception (see Valproate).
Important interactions	Phenytoin is an enzyme inducer, so reduces plasma concentrations and efficacy of ▲**drugs metabolised by P450 enzymes,** e.g. warfarin, and oestrogens and progestogens. Phenytoin is itself metabolised by these enzymes, so its plasma concentrations and adverse effects are increased by ▲**cytochrome P450 inhibitors,** e.g. amiodarone, diltiazem and fluconazole. Complex interactions can occur with ▲**other antiepileptic drugs** as most alter drug metabolism. The efficacy of antiepileptic drugs is reduced by ▲**drugs that lower the seizure threshold** (e.g. SSRIs, tricyclic antidepressants, antipsychotics, tramadol).

PRACTICAL PRESCRIBING

Prescription	**Intravenous phenytoin** is prescribed for status epilepticus at a loading dose of 20 mg/kg (max 2 g), followed by a maintenance dose of 100 mg 6–8-hrly. Long-term **oral phenytoin** for chronic epilepsy is commenced at 150–300 mg daily, in 1–2 divided doses. Phenytoin dosage is adjusted according to plasma concentrations. Treatment should **not be stopped suddenly,** but should be withdrawn gradually under medical supervision, due to risk of seizure recurrence.
Administration	**IV phenytoin** is given as a slow IV injection or infusion (maximum 50 mg/min) into a large vein. The **cannula is flushed** before and after injection using 0.9% sodium chloride to prevent venous irritation. Cardiac resuscitation facilities should be available. **Oral phenytoin** is formulated as phenytoin sodium (tablets or capsules) or phenytoin base (chewable tablets or oral solution). As phenytoin content of these formulations is not identical, plasma concentration monitoring is required if switching between preparations.
Communication	Explain that the aim of treatment is to reduce frequency of seizures. Advise the patient to take phenytoin regularly with or after food and not to miss any doses. Warn them to seek urgent medical advice for skin rashes, bruising or signs of infection (such as high temperature or sore throat), which could indicate hypersensitivity. For women, discuss contraception and pregnancy (see Valproate). Advise them not to drive unless seizure-free for 12 months (or asleep-only seizures over 3 years) and for 6 months after changing or stopping treatment.
Monitoring	**Plasma phenytoin concentrations** measured immediately before the next dose should be 10–20 mg/L. If needed, make small changes in dose (e.g. by 50 mg) at a time, as zero-order kinetics makes the effect of change difficult to predict. After a dose change, wait at least 7 days before repeating blood tests to determine new steady state plasma concentrations. Monitor **efficacy** by comparing seizure frequency before and after starting or changing treatment. Monitor blood pressure, cardiac rhythm, respiratory rate and oxygen saturations to look for **adverse effects** during IV treatment.
Cost	Phenytoin preparations vary widely in price.

Clinical tip—In elderly patients, a reduced level of consciousness can sometimes be caused by non-convulsive status epilepticus, which can be difficult to diagnose. Where electroencephalography (EEG) is not readily available, a therapeutic trial of phenytoin may be useful in confirming this differential and occasionally results in a dramatic improvement in consciousness.

Phosphodiesterase (type 5) inhibitors

CLINICAL PHARMACOLOGY

Common indications	❶ Erectile dysfunction. ❷ Primary pulmonary hypertension.
Mechanisms of action	Sildenafil is a phosphodiesterase (PDE) inhibitor. It is **selective for PDE type-5** that is found predominantly in the smooth muscle of the corpus cavernosum of the penis and arteries of the lung. For an erection to occur, sexual stimulation is required. This releases nitric oxide, which stimulates cyclic guanosine monophosphate (cGMP) production, causing arterial smooth muscle relaxation, vasodilatation and penile engorgement. As PDE5 is responsible for the breakdown of cGMP, inhibition of this enzyme by **sildenafil increases cGMP concentrations, improving penile blood flow** and **erection quality.** It is worth noting sildenafil does not cause an erection without sexual stimulation. In the pulmonary vasculature, sildenafil causes arterial vasodilatation by similar mechanisms so is used to treat **primary pulmonary hypertension.**
Important adverse effects	Most of the adverse effects of sildenafil relate to its actions as a vasodilator. These include **flushing, headache, dizziness** and **nasal congestion.** More seriously, **hypotension, tachycardia** and **palpitations** can occur and there is a small associated risk of **vascular events** (e.g. myocardial infarction, stroke). If the erection fails to subside for a prolonged period despite absence of stimulation (**priapism**), urgent medical assistance is required to prevent penile damage. **Visual disorders** including colour distortion are due to inhibition of PDE6 in the retina and should prompt urgent medical review.
Warnings	You should not prescribe sildenafil for patients in whom vasodilatation could be dangerous, including those with recent ✘**stroke** or ✘**acute coronary syndrome** or with significant history of ✘**cardiovascular disease**. Sildenafil should be avoided or used at a lower dose in people with severe ▲**hepatic** or ▲**renal impairment** in whom sildenafil metabolism and excretion is reduced.
Important interactions	Do not prescribe sildenafil for people taking any drug that increases nitric oxide, particularly ✘nitrates or ✘nicorandil, as their combined effects on cGMP (see Mechanisms of action) can cause marked arterial vasodilatation and cardiovascular collapse. Prescribe sildenafil with caution in patients taking other ▲**vasodilators** including α-blockers (should not be taken within 4 hours of sildenafil) and calcium channel blockers, as there is an increased risk of hypotension. Plasma concentrations and adverse effects of sildenafil are increased by ▲**cytochrome P450 inhibitors,** e.g. amiodarone, diltiazem and fluconazole.

PRACTICAL PRESCRIBING

Prescription	Sildenafil is available as two different preparations. **Viagra®** (available in 25 mg, 50 mg and 100 mg tablets) is used for the treatment of **erectile dysfunction.** It should be prescribed to be taken as required before sex. The usual starting dose is 50 mg orally, with a maximum of one dose per day. **Revatio®** (available as 20 mg tablets, oral suspension and for IV administration) is used for the treatment of **pulmonary hypertension**. It should be prescribed for regular administration, usually at a starting dose of 20 mg orally three times a day. Note that the different tablet strengths of the two preparations means that they cannot be used interchangeably.
Administration	Absorption of oral sildenafil and onset of effect will be delayed if it is taken with food.
Communication	For the treatment of erectile dysfunction, explain that you are prescribing a drug that will help them to have and maintain an erection, but that the **drug will not produce an erection without sexual stimulation.** Advise the patient that sildenafil should be **taken an hour before sex** to allow sufficient time for absorption. Warn them to seek medical advice if the erection does not subside within two hours after sexual activity has finished. They should also report any eyesight changes.
Monitoring	You should review the patient to enquire about therapeutic efficacy and side effects. Patients with pulmonary hypertension should have regular monitoring with a specialist.
Cost	Phosphodiesterase (type 5) inhibitors are relatively expensive. For erectile dysfunction, they can only be prescribed within the NHS where the problem is secondary to chronic disease (e.g. diabetes mellitus, Parkinson's disease) or trauma (e.g. pelvic surgery, spinal cord injury). Specialist services can prescribe sildenafil if they judge that erectile dysfunction is causing significant psychological or social stress. Sildenafil is formulated as two preparations. It is worth noting, however, that the patent for Viagra® expired in June 2013, so cheaper, non-proprietary formulations may become available in the near future.

Clinical tip—Some people take the recreational drug amyl nitrate (poppers) as an aphrodisiac. Warn them not to take this while they are on sildenafil as the combination may cause them to collapse.

Potassium, oral

CLINICAL PHARMACOLOGY

Common indications	❶ Treatment and prevention of **potassium depletion.** This is usually evident from a low serum potassium concentration (**hypokalaemia**). Addition of a drug with <u>potassium-sparing diuretic</u> effects is preferred when potassium losses are due to <u>loop-</u> or <u>thiazide-diuretic</u> therapy. <u>Intravenous potassium chloride</u> is preferred in the initial treatment of hypokalaemia that is severe (<2.5 mmol/L), symptomatic, or causing arrhythmias.
Mechanisms of action	**Hypokalaemia** is usually, although not always, due to **potassium depletion.** This may be because of, for example, diarrhoea, vomiting, or secondary hyperaldosteronism. Potassium supplementation may restore normal potassium balance in this scenario. By contrast, if losses are due to <u>loop-</u> or <u>thiazide-diuretic</u> therapy, supplementation is largely ineffective. This is because although the serum potassium concentration is low, intake and output are in balance. Potassium supplementation results simply in increased potassium excretion and only minimal effect on serum concentration. Treatment with a <u>potassium-sparing diuretic</u> (or <u>aldosterone antagonist</u>) is therefore preferred. In **redistributive hypokalaemia** the total body potassium content is normal, but the serum concentration is low because of redistribution into cells. Drug therapy (e.g. with <u>insulin</u>, <u>salbutamol</u>) is most often the culprit. Management should ideally be to address the underlying cause.
Important adverse effects	Oral potassium preparations are not very well tolerated, mainly because they are **unpalatable** and cause **gastrointestinal disturbance,** including nausea, vomiting, pain, diarrhoea and flatulence. Modified-release preparations may be better tolerated, but these can cause **gastrointestinal obstruction, ulceration** and **bleeding.** Overtreatment may lead to **hyperkalaemia** and a resultant risk of **arrhythmias.**
Warnings	Potassium supplements must be used with caution (lower dose and more intensive monitoring) in patients with ▲**renal impairment,** due to the greatly increased risk of hyperkalaemia. They should be avoided in ✖**severe renal impairment.**
Important interactions	Oral potassium supplements have additive effects with other ▲**potassium-elevating drugs,** including <u>intravenous potassium chloride</u>, <u>aldosterone antagonists</u>, <u>potassium-sparing diuretics</u>, <u>ACE inhibitors</u> and <u>angiotensin receptor blockers</u>.

potassium chloride, potassium bicarbonate

PRACTICAL PRESCRIBING

Prescription	In general, treatment is required when the serum potassium concentration falls below 3.0 mmol/L, or 3.5 mmol/L in patients at high risk of arrhythmias (e.g. those taking <u>digoxin</u>). Oral replacement is most commonly given as potassium chloride with potassium bicarbonate (e.g. Sando-K® tablets) or potassium chloride alone (e.g. Kay-Cee-L® syrup). Sando-K® contains 12 mmol of potassium per tablet; Kay-Cee-L® contains 1 mmol/mL. A typical regimen would be Sando-K® 2 tablets two or three times daily. This provides 48 or 72 mmol of potassium per day, respectively. The dose is adjusted to response.
Administration	Sando-K® is an effervescent tablet. It is stirred in about half a glassful of water for administration. Some patients find it best to take it with food.
Communication	Advise patients that they have a low level of potassium in their blood, and without treatment this could upset their heart rhythm. Ensure they understand the importance of blood test monitoring. Explain the common side effects and advise that these may be reduced by combining the doses with a meal or snack. Advise them not to consume 'salt substitutes', e.g. LoSalt®. These have high potassium content and, because the amount consumed inevitably varies, can make it difficult to get the potassium dose right.
Monitoring	At baseline, an electrocardiogram should be recorded to confirm the absence of hypokalaemic changes (e.g. small T-waves, prolonged QT interval and appearance of U-waves) and therefore suitability for oral treatment. The potassium concentration should be monitored during therapy. The frequency of monitoring is determined on a case-by-case basis, according to the severity and cause of the hypokalaemia.
Cost	Oral potassium chloride preparations are relatively inexpensive.

Clinical tip—Always beware of the risk of rebound hyperkalaemia when you are treating hypokalaemia. This is especially important if the patient has renal impairment or if there is a redistributive component to the hypokalaemia. Monitor the serum potassium concentration closely and stop potassium replacement as soon as possible.

Prostaglandin analogue eye drops

CLINICAL PHARMACOLOGY

Common indications	❶ As first-line agents to lower intraocular pressure in **open-angle glaucoma** and **ocular hypertension.** Prostaglandin analogues are generally preferred over topical β-blockers (the main alternative class) as they cause fewer systemic side effects.
Mechanisms of action	Elevated intraocular pressure **(ocular hypertension)** is a risk factor for **open-angle glaucoma.** Glaucoma is characterised by progressive optic nerve damage associated with visual field loss and eventually blindness. It is usually, although not always, associated with elevated intraocular pressure. Either way, lowering intraocular pressure reduces glaucoma progression. Analogues of prostaglandin $F_{2\alpha}$ reduce intraocular pressure by increasing outflow of aqueous humour via the uveoscleral pathway. The exact mechanism for this is uncertain.
Important adverse effects	Prostaglandin analogue eyedrops have few systemic side effects. Locally in the eye they may cause **blurred vision, conjunctival reddening (hyperaemia),** and **ocular irritation and pain.** They may also cause a **permanent change in eye colour** by increasing the amount of melanin in stromal melanocytes of the iris. This affects about one in three patients and is most noticeable when treatment is restricted to one eye.
Warnings	Caution is needed when contemplating prostaglandin analogue treatment in eyes in which the lens is absent (▲**aphakia**) or artificial (▲**pseudophakia**); and in patients with or at risk of ▲**iritis,** ▲**uveitis** or ▲**macular oedema.** In patients with **severe asthma** there is a theoretical risk of provoking bronchoconstriction, but in practice this does not seem to be a problem. It is certainly less of a concern than with topical β-blockers.
Important interactions	There are no clinically important interactions.

latanoprost, bimatoprost

PRACTICAL PRESCRIBING

Prescription	The decision to offer pharmacological treatment in **ocular hypertension** is made by a specialist, taking into account the patient's age, intraocular pressure and central corneal thickness. All patients with confirmed **open-angle glaucoma** should be offered pharmacological treatment, again by a specialist. Usually this is with latanoprost 0.005% eye drop solution, 1 drop administered to the affected eye(s) once daily.
Administration	It is best to administer latanoprost eye drops in the evening. Contact lenses should be removed before instilling the drops. They may be reinserted 15 minutes later.
Communication	Explain that the aim of treatment is to reduce the risk of sight loss. Advise patients how to administer the eye drops correctly. Warn them about the possibility of a change in eye colour. This advice may be tailored according to the patients' eye colour, since it is most likely in those with mixed-colour irides (i.e. brown plus another colour), and very rare in those with a homogenous eye colour ('pure' blue, grey, green, or brown). Explain that it is usually only slight and is not harmful, but if it occurs it is likely to be permanent.
Monitoring	Patients should be reviewed regularly by a suitably trained and experienced healthcare professional. The monitoring interval is determined according to intraocular pressure and risk of conversion to glaucoma.
Cost	Prostaglandin eye drops are relatively expensive, but with competition from non-proprietary products the cost is falling. At the time of writing, the leading latanoprost brand (Xalatan®) was about five times the price of non-proprietary latanoprost.

Clinical tip—Advice that may be given for all eye drops is that the patient should gently compress the medial canthus (the nasal 'corner') of the eye for about 1 minute, immediately after instilling the drop. This reduces systemic absorption of the drug.

Proton pump inhibitors

CLINICAL PHARMACOLOGY

Common indications	Proton pump inhibitors are a first-line treatment for: ❶ Prevention and treatment of **peptic ulcer disease,** including **NSAID-associated ulcers.** ❷ Symptomatic relief of **dyspepsia** and **gastro-oesophageal reflux disease.** ❸ Eradication of *Helicobacter pylori* **infection,** in which they are used in combination with antibiotic therapy.
Mechanisms of action	Proton pump inhibitors (PPIs) reduce gastric acid secretion. They act by **irreversibly inhibiting H⁺/K⁺-ATPase in gastric parietal cells.** This is the 'proton pump' responsible for secreting H⁺ and generating gastric acid. An advantage of targeting the final stage of gastric acid production is that they are able to suppress gastric acid production almost completely. In this respect they differ from H₂-receptor antagonists.
Important adverse effects	Common side effects of PPIs include **gastrointestinal disturbances** and **headache.** By increasing the gastric pH, PPIs may reduce the body's host defence against infection; there is some evidence of increased risk of *Clostridium difficile* infection in patients taking PPIs. Prolonged treatment with PPIs can cause **hypomagnesaemia,** which if severe can lead to tetany and ventricular arrhythmia.
Warnings	PPIs may **disguise symptoms of gastric cancer,** so prescribers should enquire about 'alarm symptoms' before and during treatment (see Communication). There is epidemiological evidence that PPIs, particularly when administered at high dose for prolonged courses in the elderly, can **increase the risk of fracture.** Patients at risk of ▲osteoporosis should therefore be identified and treated as appropriate.
Important interactions	There is some evidence that PPIs, particularly omeprazole, reduce the antiplatelet effect of ▲clopidogrel by decreasing its activation by cytochrome P450 enzymes. Understanding continues to evolve on this issue, but current evidence suggests that lansoprazole and pantoprazole have a lower propensity to interact with clopidogrel. As such, these are the preferred PPIs when prescribing alongside clopidogrel.

lansoprazole, omeprazole, pantoprazole

PRACTICAL PRESCRIBING

Prescription	Oral and injectable preparations are available. The dose of PPI depends on the drug and indication, and these are detailed in the BNF. Generally the lowest effective dose should be used for the shortest period possible. The BNF provides a helpful table of recommended regimens for *H. pylori* eradication.
Administration	Oral preparations can be taken with food or on an empty stomach. They are best taken in the morning. Intravenous preparations should be given by slow injection or infusion.
Communication	Explain that you are offering treatment to reduce stomach acid. This will hopefully improve their symptoms and, if applicable, allow their ulcer to heal. Ensure that both you and the patient are clear on the intended duration of therapy (e.g. a 7-day course to eradicate *H. pylori,* or long-term therapy to protect against ulcers) and how success will be judged (e.g. evidence of healing on endoscopy, or simply by resolution of symptoms). Ask the patient to report any problems, particularly 'alarm' symptoms (e.g. weight loss, swallowing difficulty).
Monitoring	Response to treatment should be monitored in terms of symptomatic response and, in some cases (e.g. peptic ulcers), endoscopic appearance. In prolonged use (>1 year) you should check serum magnesium levels due to the risk of hypomagnesaemia.
Cost	Relatively inexpensive non-proprietary formulations are available and should be preferred in most cases.

Clinical tip—Patients undergoing investigation for *H. pylori* infection should ideally withhold their PPI for 2 weeks before testing. This is because it increases the chance of a false negative result.

Quinine

CLINICAL PHARMACOLOGY

Common indications	❶ Quinine is commonly used for the treatment and prevention of night-time **leg cramps,** but should really be reserved for cases when cramps regularly disrupt sleep and when non-pharmacological methods, such as passive stretching exercises, have failed. ❷ Quinine is a first-line treatment option for *Plasmodium falciparum* **malaria.**
Mechanisms of action	**Leg cramps** are caused by sudden, painful involuntary contraction of skeletal muscle. Quinine is thought to act by reducing the excitability of the motor end plate in response to acetylcholine stimulation. This reduces the frequency of muscle contraction. In **malaria,** the mechanism of action of quinine is not well understood, but its overall effect leads to rapid killing of *P. falciparum* parasites in the schizont stage in the blood.
Important adverse effects	Although quinine is usually safe at recommended doses, it is potentially very toxic and can be fatal in overdose. It can cause **tinnitus, deafness** and **blindness** (which may be permanent), **gastrointestinal upset,** and **hypersensitivity** reactions. Quinine **prolongs the QT interval,** and may therefore predispose to arrhythmias. **Hypoglycaemia** can occur and can be particularly problematic in patients with malaria, which also predisposes to hypoglycaemia.
Warnings	Quinine should be prescribed with caution in people with existing ▲**hearing or visual loss.** It is **teratogenic,** so should not be prescribed in the ▲**first trimester** of pregnancy, although in the case of malaria its benefit may outweigh this risk. Quinine should be avoided in people with ▲**G6PD deficiency,** as it can precipitate haemolysis.
Important interactions	Quinine should be prescribed with caution in patients taking other ▲**drugs that prolong the QT interval** or cause arrhythmias such as amiodarone, antipsychotics, quinolones, macrolides, and SSRIs.

PRACTICAL PRESCRIBING

Prescription	For nocturnal **leg cramps,** quinine should be prescribed for oral administration at a dose of 200–300 mg, to be taken at night. In the treatment of **malaria,** higher doses of quinine are required. It may be prescribed to be taken orally for uncomplicated cases (alongside another antimalarial medication such as <u>doxycycline</u>) or for IV administration in severe cases. Intravenous dosing should be based on the patient's weight.
Administration	IV quinine should be given as a slow infusion.
Communication	For nocturnal **leg cramps,** explain that you are recommending a 4-week trial of quinine in the hope of reducing the frequency of cramps. Explain that if there is no improvement after 4 weeks they are unlikely to experience any benefit and should stop taking it. Ask your patient to report any adverse effects, such as hearing loss, visual disturbance and palpitations immediately, as quinine is potentially harmful to the ears, eyes and heart.
Monitoring	Review your patient's symptoms after 4 weeks and advise them to stop taking quinine if there has not been a significant improvement. If you decide to continue treatment, review them again at 3 months and consider a trial discontinuation at that stage. Aim to avoid long-term use due to the potential for serious adverse effects.
Cost	Quinine sulfate is available in non-proprietary formulations and is relatively inexpensive.

Clinical tip—Although quinine is commonly prescribed for people with nocturnal leg cramps, its benefit is relatively modest, reducing the frequency of cramps only by around 20%. Before starting treatment, you should first exclude reversible causes, such as electrolyte disturbances and drug causes (e.g. <u>statins</u>, <u>β₂-agonists</u>), and attempt non-pharmacological treatments such as passive stretching exercises. If you do decide to start treatment, review your patient after a month; if they have not experienced any significant benefit then consider stopping treatment.

Quinolones

CLINICAL PHARMACOLOGY

Common indications	Quinolones are generally reserved as second or third-line treatment due to the potential for rapid emergence of resistance and an association with *Clostridium difficile* infection. With these caveats in mind, they are used in: ❶ **Urinary tract infection (UTI).** ❷ **Severe gastrointestinal infection,** e.g. with *Shigella, Campylobacter*. ❸ **Lower respiratory tract infection (LRTI)** (moxifloxacin, levofloxacin). ❹ Ciprofloxacin is the only oral antibiotic in common use with activity against **Pseudomonas aeruginosa.** Moxifloxacin and levofloxacin do not have this property.
Mechanisms of action	Quinolones kill bacteria by **inhibiting DNA synthesis.** They are particularly active against aerobic Gram-negative bacteria, which explains their utility in treatment of urinary and gastrointestinal infections. Moxifloxacin and levofloxacin are newer quinolones with enhanced activity against Gram-positive organisms. They can therefore be used to treat LRTI, which may be caused by either Gram-positive or Gram-negative organisms. **Bacteria rapidly develop resistance** to quinolones. Some bacteria prevent intracellular accumulation of the drug by reducing permeability and/or increasing efflux. Others develop protective mutations in target enzymes. Quinolone resistance genes are spread horizontally between bacteria by plasmids, accelerating acquisition of resistance.
Important adverse effects	Quinolones are generally well tolerated although they can cause **gastrointestinal upset** (including nausea and diarrhoea) and immediate and delayed **hypersensitivity** reactions. Class-specific adverse reactions include **neurological effects** (lowering of the seizure threshold and hallucinations), and inflammation and **rupture of muscle tendons.** Quinolones (particularly moxifloxacin) **prolong the QT interval** and therefore increase the risk of **arrhythmias.** They promote *Clostridium difficile* **colitis,** particularly with the hypervirulent 027 strain.
Warnings	Quinolones should be used with caution in people at particular risk of adverse effects including those ▲**with or at risk of seizures,** ▲**who are growing** (potential risk of arthropathy); and with other ▲**risk factors for QT prolongation** (such as cardiac disease or electrolyte disturbance).
Important interactions	Drugs containing divalent cations (e.g. <u>calcium</u>, <u>antacids</u>) reduce absorption and efficacy of quinolones. Ciprofloxacin inhibits certain cytochrome P450 enzymes, increasing risk of toxicity with some drugs, notably ▲**theophylline.** Co-prescription of <u>NSAIDs</u> increases the risk of **seizures,** and of <u>prednisolone</u> increases the risk of **tendon rupture.** Quinolones should be prescribed with caution in patients taking other ▲**drugs that prolong the QT interval** or cause arrhythmias, such as <u>amiodarone</u>, <u>antipsychotics</u>, <u>quinine</u>, <u>macrolide antibiotics</u> and <u>SSRIs</u>.

PRACTICAL PRESCRIBING

Prescription	Quinolones are rapidly and extensively absorbed in the intestine, so **high plasma concentrations** can be achieved by **oral administration.** Intravenous prescription should therefore usually be reserved for people unable to take drugs by mouth or absorb them in the intestine (also see Cost). They are eliminated by the kidney and have relatively long plasma half-lives, so are administered every 12–24 hours. Typical dosages are: *ciprofloxacin* 250–750 mg orally 12-hrly or 400 mg IV 12-hrly; *moxifloxacin* 400 mg oral/IV daily; and *levofloxacin* 500 mg oral/IV daily. Duration of therapy is determined by the type and severity of infection.
Administration	Oral quinolones are available as tablets, with ciprofloxacin also being formulated as a (more expensive) oral suspension. Intravenous quinolones come pre-prepared in solution for infusion over 60 minutes.
Communication	Explain that the aim of treatment is to get rid of infection and improve symptoms. For oral treatment, encourage the patient to complete the prescribed course. Before prescribing, always check with your patient personally or get collateral history to ensure that they do not have an **allergy** to quinolones (any 'floxacin'). Warn them to seek medical advice if a rash or other unexpected symptoms develop. If an allergy develops during treatment, give the patient written and verbal advice not to take this antibiotic in the future and make sure that the allergy is clearly documented in their medical records.
Monitoring	Check that infection resolves by resolution of symptoms, signs (e.g. pyrexia, lung crackles) and blood markers (e.g. falling C-reactive protein and white cell count) as appropriate.
Cost	Ciprofloxacin currently costs around 10p for a 500 mg tablet and around £20 (with additional administration costs) for a 400 mg infusion.

Clinical tip—Ciprofloxacin has good antibacterial activity against organisms causing severe traveller's diarrhoea, including shigella, salmonella and campylobacter. You could ask your GP for a pack to take on elective study trips to remote high-risk destinations! However, antibiotics should be reserved for severe infection (e.g. with systemic involvement) as use in milder infections will have little clinical benefit and increase the risk of resistance.

Statins

CLINICAL PHARMACOLOGY

Common indications	❶ **Primary prevention of cardiovascular disease:** to prevent cardiovascular events in people over 40 years of age with a 10-year cardiovascular risk >20%. ❷ **Secondary prevention of cardiovascular disease:** first line alongside lifestyle changes, to prevent further cardiovascular events in those who already have evidence of cardiovascular disease. ❸ **Primary hyperlipidaemia:** first line, in conditions such as primary hypercholesterolaemia, mixed dyslipidaemia and familial hypercholesterolaemia.
Mechanisms of action	Statins reduce serum cholesterol levels. They **inhibit 3-hydroxy-3-methyl-glutaryl coenzyme A (HMG CoA) reductase,** an enzyme involved in making cholesterol. They decrease cholesterol production by the liver and increase clearance of LDL-cholesterol from the blood, reducing LDL-cholesterol levels. They also indirectly reduce triglycerides and slightly increase HDL-cholesterol levels. Through these effects they slow the atherosclerotic process and may even reverse it.
Important adverse effects	Statins are generally safe and well tolerated. The most common adverse effects are **headache** and **gastrointestinal disturbances.** Potentially more serious are their effects on muscle. These can range from simple **aches** to more serious **myopathy** or, rarely, **rhabdomyolysis.** They can also cause a **rise in liver enzymes** (e.g. alanine transaminase [ALT]); drug-induced hepatitis is a rare but serious adverse effect.
Warnings	Statins should be used with caution in patients with existing ▲**hepatic impairment.** They are excreted by the kidneys, so the dose should be reduced in people with ▲**renal impairment.** You should avoid prescribing statins to women who are ▲**pregnant** (cholesterol is essential for normal fetal development) or ▲**breastfeeding.**
Important interactions	The metabolism of statins is reduced by ▲**cytochrome P450 inhibitors,** such as <u>amiodarone</u>, <u>diltiazem</u>, <u>itraconazole</u>, <u>macrolides</u> and protease inhibitors. This leads to accumulation of the statin in the body, which may put patients at increased risk of adverse effects. ▲<u>Amlodipine</u> has a similar interaction although the mechanism is less clear. To reduce this risk you may need to reduce the dose of the statin or, if the other drug is being used for a short period only (e.g. a course of clarithromycin therapy), withhold the statin.

simvastatin, atorvastatin, pravastatin, rosuvastatin

PRACTICAL PRESCRIBING

Prescription	Statins are taken **orally** on a once daily basis. A typical starting dose in primary prevention is simvastatin 40 mg daily or atorvastatin 10 mg daily. Higher doses may be used for secondary prevention.
Administration	Statins are traditionally taken in the **evening,** as there is some evidence that they have a greater effect when dietary intake is at its lowest.
Communication	Explain you are prescribing a medicine to lower cholesterol levels to reduce the risk of a heart attack or stroke in the future. Advise patients of common side effects, and to seek medical attention if they experience **muscle symptoms** (e.g. pain or weakness). Ask your patient to come back for **blood tests** in 3 and 12 months. Advise them to keep alcohol intake to a minimum. Those taking simvastatin or atorvastatin should **avoid grapefruit juice,** which inhibits the cytochrome P450 enzymes that metabolise statins and may therefore increase the risk of side effects. This is not the case for pravastatin and rosuvastatin.
Monitoring	In **primary prevention** of cardiovascular disease, you should check a lipid profile before treatment but thereafter this does not need to be checked routinely, as there are no specified target levels in current guidelines. However, the inverse of this is true in **secondary prevention.** A baseline lipid profile is not necessary in patients with established cardiovascular disease, but **efficacy** should be monitored by checking target cholesterol levels are achieved, as specified in guidelines. If these are not achieved you could consider switching to an alternative statin or a different class of lipid-lowering agent. For **safety,** check liver enzymes (e.g. ALT) at baseline and again at 3 and 12 months. A rise in ALT up to three times the upper limit of normal may be acceptable but above this should lead to discontinuation. The statin can be restarted at a lower dose when liver enzymes have returned to normal. You do not need to check creatine kinase routinely, but you should ask patients to report muscle symptoms.
Cost	Statins that are available in non-proprietary form (e.g. simvastatin, atorvastatin) are inexpensive, and should be preferred over branded products.

Clinical tip—Do not forget to check a patient's thyroid function before starting a statin. Hypothyroidism is a reversible cause of hyperlipidaemia, and should therefore be corrected before reassessing the need for lipid-lowering medications. Furthermore, hypothyroidism increases the risk of myositis with statins.

Sulphonylureas

CLINICAL PHARMACOLOGY

Common indications	❶ **Type 2 diabetes mellitus:** As a *single agent* to control blood glucose and reduce complications where <u>metformin</u> is contraindicated or not tolerated. In *combination* with metformin (and/or other hypoglycaemic agents) where blood glucose is not adequately controlled on a single agent.
Mechanisms of action	Sulphonylureas lower blood glucose by **stimulating pancreatic insulin secretion.** They block ATP-dependent K^+ channels in pancreatic β-cell membranes, causing depolarisation of the cell membrane and opening of voltage-gated Ca^{2+} channels. This increases intracellular Ca^{2+} concentrations, stimulating insulin secretion. Sulphonylureas are only effective in patients with residual pancreatic function. As insulin is an anabolic hormone, stimulation of insulin secretion by sulphonylureas is associated with weight gain. Weight gain increases insulin resistance and can worsen diabetes mellitus in the long term.
Important adverse effects	Dose-related side effects such as **gastrointestinal upset** (nausea, vomiting, diarrhoea, constipation) are usually mild and infrequent. **Hypoglycaemia** is a potentially serious adverse effect, which is more likely with high treatment doses, where drug metabolism is reduced (see Warnings) or where other hypoglycaemic medications are prescribed (see Important interactions). Sulphonylurea-induced hypoglycaemia may last for many hours and, if severe, should be managed in hospital. **Rare hypersensitivity reactions** include hepatic toxicity (e.g. cholestatic jaundice), drug hypersensitivity syndrome (rash, fever, internal organ involvement) and haematological abnormalities (e.g. agranulocytosis).
Warnings	Gliclazide is metabolised in the liver and has a plasma half-life of 10–12 hours. Unchanged drug and metabolites are excreted in the urine. A dose reduction may therefore be required in patients with ▲**hepatic impairment** and blood glucose should be monitored carefully in patients with ▲**renal impairment.** Sulphonylureas should be prescribed with caution for people at ▲**increased risk of hypoglycaemia,** including those with hepatic impairment (reduced gluconeogenesis), malnutrition, adrenal or pituitary insufficiency (lack of counter-regulatory hormones) and the elderly.
Important interactions	Risk of hypoglycaemia is increased by co-prescription of other antidiabetic drugs including <u>metformin</u>, <u>thiazolidinediones</u> (e.g. pioglitazone) and <u>insulin</u>. The efficacy of sulphonylureas is reduced by drugs that elevate blood glucose, e.g. <u>prednisolone</u>, <u>thiazide</u> and <u>loop diuretics</u>.

PRACTICAL PRESCRIBING

Prescription	There are several sulphonylureas to choose from. Those with a shorter duration of action and hepatic metabolism (e.g. gliclazide) are the easiest to use, particularly in elderly patients with impaired renal function. Sulphonylureas are prescribed for oral administration only. Gliclazide (standard release) is usually started at a dosage of 40–80 mg once daily. The dose is increased gradually until blood glucose is controlled, with higher doses (160–320 mg daily) being given as two divided doses. Gliclazide is also formulated as a modified-release form. Note that the 80 mg standard-release tablets contain the same amount of gliclazide as the 30 mg modified-release tablets. It is important to prescribe these carefully to avoid dosing errors. Sulphonylureas are a long-term treatment that in general should be stopped or changed only if adverse effects are intolerable or new contraindications develop.
Administration	Sulphonylureas should be taken with meals (e.g. once daily at breakfast or twice daily at breakfast and evening meal).
Communication	Advise patients that a sulphonylurea has been prescribed to control the blood sugar level and reduce the risk of diabetic complications, such as heart attacks. Explain that tablets are not a replacement for **lifestyle measures** and should be taken in addition to a calorie-controlled diet and regular exercise. Warn them about **hypoglycaemia,** advising them to watch out for symptoms, such as dizziness, nausea, sweating and confusion. If hypoglycaemia develops, they should take something sugary (e.g. glucose tablets or a sugary drink) then something starchy (e.g. a sandwich), and seek medical advice if symptoms recur.
Monitoring	Assess blood glucose control by measuring **glycated haemoglobin (HbA$_{1c}$)** (target <58 mmol/mol). Blood glucose monitoring is not routinely required, although measurement may be helpful to determine if any unusual symptoms are due to hypoglycaemia. Measurement of renal and hepatic function before treatment can determine need for caution or identify contraindications to treatment.
Cost	Non-proprietary gliclazide 80 mg tablets cost as little as 2.5p each. This is considerably cheaper than newer antidiabetic drugs, e.g. exenatide and sitagliptin, which cost £1–£2 per dose.

Clinical tip—During acute illness, insulin resistance increases and renal and hepatic function may become impaired. All oral hypoglycaemics become less effective at controlling blood glucose and side effects are more likely, e g hypoglycaemia with sulphonylureas. In hospital inpatients, insulin treatment may be required temporarily during severe illness. Insulin has a short half-life and its dosage can be adjusted more easily than with oral medication in response to acute fluctuations in blood glucose.

Tetracyclines

CLINICAL PHARMACOLOGY

Common indications	❶ **Acne vulgaris,** particularly where there are inflamed papules, pustules and/or cysts (*Proprionibacterium acnes*). ❷ **Lower respiratory tract infections** including **infective exacerbations of COPD** (e.g. *Haemophilus influenzae*), **pneumonia** and **atypical pneumonia** (mycoplasma, *Chlamydia psittaci*, *Coxiella burnetii* [Q fever]). ❸ Chlamydial infection including **pelvic inflammatory disease.** ❹ Other infections such as typhoid, anthrax, malaria and Lyme disease (*Borrelia burgdorferi*).
Mechanisms of action	Tetracyclines **inhibit bacterial protein synthesis.** They bind to the ribosomal 30S subunit found specifically in bacteria. This prevents binding of transfer RNA to messenger RNA, which prevents addition of new amino acids to growing polypeptide chains. Inhibition of protein synthesis is 'bacteriostatic' (stops bacterial growth), which assists the immune system in killing and removing bacteria from the body. Tetracyclines have a relatively broad spectrum of antibacterial activity. Tetracyclines were discovered in 1945 and have been widely used. Consequently, some bacteria have acquired resistance to these antibiotics. A common mechanism is through acquisition of an efflux pump, which allows bacteria to pump out tetracyclines, preventing cytoplasmic accumulation.
Important adverse effects	Like most antibiotics, tetracyclines commonly cause **nausea, vomiting** and **diarrhoea,** although they are considered to be among the lowest risk antibiotics for *Clostridium difficile* infection (see Penicillins, broad-spectrum). **Hypersensitivity reactions** occur in ~1% people who take tetracyclines, including immediate and delayed (see Penicillins). As antibiotic structures are different, there is no cross-reactivity with penicillins or other β-lactam antibiotics. Tetracycline-specific side effects include: **oesophageal** irritation, ulceration and dysphagia; **photosensitivity** (an exaggerated sunburn reaction when skin is exposed to light); and **discolouration** and/or hypoplasia of **tooth enamel** if prescribed for children. **Intracranial hypertension** is a rare adverse effect causing headache and visual disturbance.
Warnings	Tetracyclines bind to teeth and bones during fetal development, infancy and early childhood and so should not be prescribed during ✖**pregnancy,** ✖**breastfeeding** or for ✖**children ≤12 years of age.** They should be avoided in people with ▲**renal impairment** as their anti-anabolic effects can raise plasma urea and reduced excretion can increase the risk of adverse effects.
Important interactions	Tetracyclines bind to divalent cations. They should therefore not be given within 2 hours of calcium, antacids or iron, which will prevent antibiotic absorption. Tetracyclines can enhance the anticoagulant effect of warfarin by killing normal gut flora that synthesise vitamin K.

PRACTICAL PRESCRIBING

Prescription	Tetracyclines are only available for oral administration. The dose and frequency of administration vary between individual drugs, e.g. *doxycycline* 100–200 mg orally daily, *lymecycline* 408–816 mg orally 12-hrly. As with other antibiotics, higher doses are prescribed for more severe or difficult to treat infections. The duration of treatment depends on the indication; for example, 5–7 days in **infective exacerbations of COPD,** 8 weeks in **acne.**
Administration	Tetracyclines are usually formulated as capsules or tablets. These should be swallowed whole with plenty of water while sitting or standing to stop them getting stuck in the oesophagus where they may cause ulceration.
Communication	Explain that the aim of treatment is to get rid of infection and improve symptoms. For oral treatment, encourage the patient to complete the prescribed course. Before prescribing, always check with your patient personally or get collateral history to ensure they have no **allergy** to tetracyclines. Warn them to seek medical advice if a rash or other unexpected symptoms develop. If an allergy develops during treatment, give the patient written and verbal advice not to take this antibiotic in the future and make sure that the allergy is clearly documented in their medical records.
Monitoring	Check that infection resolves by resolution of symptoms, signs (e.g. reduction in inflamed papules, pustules and cysts in acne) and blood markers (e.g. resolution of inflammatory markers in respiratory infection) as appropriate.
Cost	Tetracyclines are inexpensive. For example, a 1-week course of doxycycline 100 mg for respiratory infection costs around £1.

Clinical tip—Tetracyclines can cause nausea and vomiting when taken on an empty stomach, which can be reduced by taking these antibiotics with food. However, tetracyclines should not be taken with dairy products as calcium in the gastrointestinal tract binds tetracyclines and prevents their absorption.

Thiazolidinediones

CLINICAL PHARMACOLOGY

Common indications	**❶ Type 2 diabetes mellitus:** As a *single agent* in overweight patients where metformin is contraindicated or not tolerated. Added as a *second agent* to <u>metformin</u> or a <u>sulphonylurea</u> where blood glucose control is inadequate on one drug and the metformin/sulphonylurea combination is contraindicated or not tolerated. Added as a *third agent* with metformin and a sulphonylurea where blood glucose control is inadequate as an alternative to starting <u>insulin</u>.
Mechanisms of action	Thiazolidinediones are **insulin sensitisers.** They lower blood glucose by activating the gamma subclass of nuclear peroxisome proliferator-activated receptors **(PPARγ).** This induces genes which enhance insulin action in skeletal muscle, adipose tissue and the liver, with increased peripheral glucose uptake and utilisation and reduced hepatic gluconeogenesis. Thiazolidinediones do not stimulate pancreatic insulin secretion, hence do not cause hypoglycaemia. However, they cause **weight gain,** which can increase insulin resistance.
Important adverse effects	Adverse effects of pioglitazone include **gastrointestinal upset, anaemia** and minor **neurological** effects such as dizziness, headache and disturbed vision. More serious side effects include **oedema** and **cardiac failure,** particularly where pioglitazone is prescribed with <u>insulin</u>. Pioglitazone is associated with a small increase in the risk of **bladder cancer** and an increase in **bone fractures** in women. Idiosyncratic reactions include **severe liver toxicity.** Pioglitazone is the only thiazolidinedione currently available for prescription in the UK. The marketing authorisation (license) for rosiglitazone has been suspended as cardiovascular risk associated with this drug appears greater than its potential benefits. Troglitazone was withdrawn from the market due to liver toxicity.
Warnings	Pioglitazone should be avoided or prescribed with caution in people at increased risk of serious adverse effects. It is contraindicated in people with ✖**heart failure** and should be used with caution in ▲**cardiovascular disease.** It is contraindicated if there is known ✖**bladder cancer** or macroscopic haematuria and should be used with caution in people with ▲**risk factors for bladder cancer** (e.g. smoking, occupational exposure, prior pelvic irradiation). Careful consideration should be given when prescribing pioglitazone for ▲**elderly patients,** who tend to have increased risk of cardiac disease, bladder cancer and bone fractures. Pioglitazone is extensively metabolised in the liver and can cause liver toxicity, so should be used with caution in ▲**hepatic impairment.**
Important interactions	Pioglitazone is usually prescribed in combination with other <u>antidiabetic drugs</u>, which increases the risk of adverse effects, e.g. hypoglycaemia and cardiac failure. There are no other significant drug interactions.

PRACTICAL PRESCRIBING

Prescription	Pioglitazone is only available for oral administration. A typical starting dose is 15–30 mg once daily with breakfast, increased to a maximum of 45 mg daily depending on response. Pioglitazone is a long-term treatment that in general should be stopped or changed only if adverse effects are intolerable or new contraindications develop.
Administration	Pioglitazone tablets should usually be taken in the morning with a glass of water. They can be taken with or without food.
Communication	Advise patients that this medicine has been prescribed to control the blood sugar level and **reduce the risk of diabetic complications,** such as heart attacks. Explain that tablets are not a replacement for **lifestyle measures** and should be taken in addition to a calorie-controlled diet and regular exercise. Warn them to seek medical advice if they develop **unexpected side effects,** including nausea, loss of appetite, lethargy and dark urine (liver toxicity), ankle swelling and difficulty breathing (heart failure), or pain, urgency or blood on passing urine (bladder cancer).
Monitoring	Monitor efficacy by measuring **glycated haemoglobin** (HbA_{1c}) before and 3–6 months after commencing treatment to determine blood glucose control. Treatment should be stopped and alternatives considered if there is no fall in HbA_{1c}. For safety, **liver enzymes** should be measured prior to and during therapy. Treatment should not be started if baseline transaminase levels are increased and may need to be discontinued if values are persistently elevated during treatment.
Cost	Pioglitazone is often combined with metformin. Monthly treatment costs are around £5 where the two drugs are prescribed separately or around £36 for the same drugs prescribed as a combination pill. Although combination pills have potential to improve treatment adherence, the likely benefit should be weighed carefully against increased costs before prescribing.

Clinical tip—Newer classes of antidiabetic agents include dipeptidyl peptidase 4-inhibitors (e.g. sitagliptin) and glucagon-like peptide-1 (GLP-1) receptor activators (e.g. exenatide). Both classes reduce blood glucose by increasing insulin and inhibiting glucagon secretion. GLP-1 agonists also slow gastric emptying. These drugs have a similar place in therapy as, and are an alternative to, pioglitazone, particularly in obese patients, in whom they promote weight loss.

Thyroid hormones

CLINICAL PHARMACOLOGY

Common indications	❶ Primary hypothyroidism. ❷ Hypothyroidism secondary to hypopituitarism.
Mechanisms of action	The thyroid gland produces thyroxine (T₄), which is converted to the more active triiodothyronine (T₃) in target tissues. Thyroid hormones **regulate metabolism and growth.** Deficiency of these hormones causes hypothyroidism, with clinical features including lethargy, weight gain, constipation and slowing of mental processes. Hypothyroidism is treated by long-term replacement of thyroid hormones, most usually as **levothyroxine** (synthetic T₄). **Liothyronine** (synthetic T₃) has a shorter half-life and quicker onset (a few hours) and offset (24–48 hours) of action than levothyroxine. It is therefore reserved for emergency treatment of severe or acute hypothyroidism.
Important adverse effects	The adverse effects of levothyroxine are usually due to excessive doses, so are predictably similar to symptoms of hyperthyroidism. These include **gastrointestinal** (e.g. diarrhoea, vomiting, weight loss), **cardiac** (e.g. palpitations, arrhythmias, angina) and **neurological** (e.g. tremor, restlessness, insomnia) manifestations.
Warnings	Thyroid hormones increase heart rate and metabolism. They can therefore precipitate cardiac ischaemia in people with ▲**coronary artery disease,** in whom replacement should be started cautiously at a low dose and with careful monitoring. In ▲**hypopituitarism,** corticosteroid therapy must be initiated before thyroid hormone replacement to avoid precipitating an Addisonian crisis.
Important interactions	As gastrointestinal absorption of levothyroxine is reduced by antacids, calcium or iron salts, administration of these drugs needs to be separated by about 4 hours. An increase in levothyroxine dose may be required in patients taking **cytochrome P450 inducers,** e.g. phenytoin, carbamazepine. Levothyroxine-induced changes in metabolism can increase insulin or oral hypoglycaemic requirements in diabetes mellitus and enhance the effects of warfarin.

PRACTICAL PRESCRIBING

Prescription	*Levothyroxine* is only available for oral administration. A starting dose of 50–100 micrograms daily is recommended, except in the elderly or people with cardiac disease, who should start on 25 micrograms daily. The dose is adjusted monthly in 25–50-microgram increments according to monitoring (see below) to a usual maintenance dose of 50–200 micrograms once daily. Remember to write micrograms in full to reduce the risk of dosing errors. *Liothyronine* is available for IV administration in emergency care. It should be prescribed only after consultation with senior and specialist colleagues.
Administration	Levothyroxine is available in 25, 50 and 100 microgram tablets, so a combination is often required for adequate dosing (e.g. patients requiring 175 micrograms will need to take one of each strength daily).
Communication	Explain that treatment will **replace a natural hormone** that their body has stopped making and that this will give them more energy and make them feel better. Advise them that it may take some time (months in some cases) for them to feel 'back to normal'. It is important to emphasise (for most people) that **treatment is for life** and that they should not stop taking it. **Warn them of the signs of too much treatment** (e.g. shakiness, anxiety, sleeplessness, diarrhoea) and advise them to see a doctor if these occur, as their treatment may need to be reduced. If they take **calcium or iron replacement,** advise them to leave a gap of about 4 hours between these treatments and levothyroxine.
Monitoring	The aim of therapy is to relieve symptoms and return the patient to a euthyroid state. Initially you should review your patient monthly and dose changes should be guided by symptoms. **Thyroid function tests** should be measured 3 months after starting treatment or a change in dose. In primary hypothyroidism, **thyroid stimulating hormone (TSH)** is the main guide to dosing. It is elevated due to loss of negative feedback of T_4 on the pituitary. With adequate levothyroxine replacement, TSH should return to normal or low-normal concentrations. Stable patients should have annual clinical review and thyroid function tests.
Cost	Non-proprietary levothyroxine treatment costs around £4 per month.

Clinical tip—Patients may experience *hyper*thyroid symptoms (see Important adverse effects) soon after they begin taking levothyroxine. If this happens, continue therapy at a lower dose (rather than stopping it) and arrange to review the patient over the next 1–2 weeks to look for the re-emergence of *hypo*thyroid symptoms. Thyroid function tests will be unhelpful in guiding therapy at this early stage as it is likely that both TSH and T_4 concentrations will be raised: TSH because the levels of this hormone take some time to normalise (weeks) and T_4 because of the levothyroxine therapy.

Trimethoprim

CLINICAL PHARMACOLOGY

Common indications	**❶** *Trimethoprim* is a first choice for uncomplicated **urinary tract infections** (UTI). Alternatives include <u>nitrofurantoin</u> and <u>amoxicillin</u>. **❷** *Co-trimoxazole* (trimethoprim combined with sulfamethoxazole) is used for treatment and prevention of **pneumocystis pneumonia** in people with immunosuppression, e.g. due to HIV infection.
Mechanisms of action	Bacteria are unable to use external sources of folate, so need to make their own for essential functions including DNA synthesis. *Trimethoprim* **inhibits bacterial folate synthesis,** slowing bacterial growth (bacteriostatic). It has a broad spectrum of action against Gram-positive and Gram-negative bacteria, particularly enterobacteria, e.g. *Escherichia coli*. However, its clinical utility is reduced by **widespread bacterial resistance.** Mechanisms of resistance include reduced intracellular antibiotic accumulation and reduced sensitivity of target enzymes. *Sulfonamides* (e.g. sulfamethoxazole) also inhibit bacterial folate synthesis, but at a different step in the pathway to trimethoprim. Together trimethoprim and sulfamethoxazole cause more complete inhibition of folate synthesis (at least *in vitro),* making them bactericidal.
Important adverse effects	Trimethoprim most commonly causes **gastrointestinal upset** (nausea, vomiting and sore mouth) and **skin rash** (3–7%). Severe **hypersensitivity** reactions, including anaphylaxis, drug fever and erythema multiforme, occur rarely with trimethoprim, but more commonly with sulfonamides, which limits their use. As a folate antagonist, trimethoprim can impair haematopoiesis, causing **haematological disorders** such as megaloblastic anaemia, leucopenia and thrombocytopenia. It can also cause **hyperkalaemia** and elevation of plasma creatinine concentrations.
Warnings	Trimethoprim is contraindicated in the ✖**first trimester of pregnancy,** because, as a folate antagonist, it is associated with an increased risk of fetal abnormalities (e.g. cardiovascular defects, oral clefts). It should be used cautiously in people with ▲**folate deficiency,** who are more susceptible to adverse haematological effects. As trimethoprim is mostly excreted unchanged into urine, it is useful in the treatment of urinary tract infections, but is less suitable in ▲**renal impairment;** if it is used, a dose reduction is necessary. ▲**Neonates,** ▲**the elderly** and people with ▲**HIV infection** are particularly susceptible to adverse effects.
Important interactions	Use with ▲**potassium-elevating drugs** (e.g. <u>aldosterone antagonists</u>, <u>ACE inhibitors</u>, <u>angiotensin receptor blockers</u>) predisposes to hyperkalaemia. Use with other **folate antagonists** (e.g. <u>methotrexate</u>) and **drugs that increase folate metabolism** (e.g. <u>phenytoin</u>) increases the risk of adverse haematological effects. Trimethoprim can enhance the anticoagulant effect of warfarin by killing normal gut flora that synthesise vitamin K.

PRACTICAL PRESCRIBING

Prescription	*Trimethoprim* is only available for oral administration. For **treatment of acute UTI** it is usually prescribed at a dosage of 200 mg 12-hrly, with duration of treatment being determined by severity of infection. As **prophylaxis for recurrent UTI,** trimethoprim is usually prescribed at a lower dose (100 mg) less often (once at night) for a prolonged period. *Co-trimoxazole* is available for oral or IV administration. The strength describes the content of both drugs, e.g. 480 mg co-trimoxazole contains 80 mg trimethoprim and 400 mg sulfamethoxazole. A weight-based dosage (120 mg/kg daily in 2–4 divided doses) is given for 14–21 days to treat **pneumocystis infection.** A lower dose (e.g. 960 mg three times a week) is used for pneumocystis prophylaxis.
Administration	Oral trimethoprim and co-trimoxazole are available as tablets and in suspension. Intravenous co-trimoxazole must be diluted immediately before use (to prevent crystallisation) in 125–500 mL sodium chloride 0.9% or glucose 5% and infused slowly over 60–90 minutes.
Communication	Explain that the aim of treatment is to get rid of infection and improve symptoms. Encourage the patient to complete the prescribed course. Before prescribing, always check with your patient personally or get collateral history to ensure that they have no **allergy** to trimethoprim or Septrin® (the brand name for co-trimoxazole). As allergic reactions are common with these antibiotics, it is particularly important to warn them to seek medical advice if a rash or other unexpected symptoms develop. If an allergy develops during treatment, give the patient written and verbal advice not to take this antibiotic in the future and make sure that the allergy is clearly documented in their medical records.
Monitoring	Check that **acute infection** resolves by resolution of symptoms (e.g. reduction in dysuria), signs (e.g. resolution of pyrexia) and investigations (e.g. fall in inflammatory markers, sterile urine on repeat culture in selected cases) as appropriate. For **long-term treatment,** full blood count monitoring may be useful for early detection and treatment of haematological disorders (e.g. by replacing folate and/or stopping the antibiotic).
Cost	Both trimethoprim and co-trimoxazole have been on the market for many years and are inexpensive.

Clinical tip—Trimethoprim competitively inhibits creatinine secretion by the renal tubules. This commonly leads to a **small reversible rise in serum creatinine concentration** during trimethoprim treatment, without reduction in the glomerular filtration rate. For this reason, trimethoprim tends to be less effective for UTI in patients with renal impairment as it is out-competed by creatinine for secretion into the urinary tract.

Vaccines

CLINICAL PHARMACOLOGY

Common indications	❶ *Childhood vaccines* are routinely offered to all children as part of the **childhood immunisation schedule.** ❷ *Influenza vaccine* is offered **annually in at-risk groups** including people aged over 6 months with chronic respiratory, heart, liver, renal or neurological disease; diabetes mellitus; immunosuppression; or HIV. ❸ *Pneumococcal vaccine* forms part of the **childhood immunisation schedule.** It is also offered for *once-only* **administration in at-risk groups.** These are similar to the at-risk groups for influenza vaccine, but with the addition of patients aged over 65 years and those with other risk factors for pneumococcal disease (cochlear implant, risk factors for cerebrospinal fluid leakage, history of invasive pneumococcal disease, occupational exposure to metal fumes and absence of a functional spleen).
Mechanisms of action	Vaccination involves administration of an antigen to **incite an adaptive immune response and generate an immune 'memory,'** usually in the form of memory B cells. This facilitates a more rapid and specific immune response on re-exposure to the antigen, attenuating the severity of infection and often rendering it subclinical. The antigen in vaccines may be provided as an **inactivated** form of the infectious agent (e.g. as in the *influenza vaccine*); a **live but attenuated** form of the infectious agent (e.g. *measles, mumps and rubella* [MMR] *vaccine*); specific protein or peptide **components** of the infectious agent (e.g. *pneumococcal vaccine*); or as a detoxified form of the **exotoxin** that would usually be produced by the infectious agent (e.g. *tetanus toxoid vaccine*).
Important adverse effects	Vaccines are very safe. The most common side effects are **local reactions** comprising pain, swelling and redness; and mild systemic effects such as **fever, headache** and **myalgia.** The MMR vaccine may cause a mild **measles-like illness** (including a rash) about 1 week after vaccination, and occasionally a **mumps-like illness** (with parotid swelling) in the third week. Very rarely, vaccines may cause severe hypersensitivity reactions including **anaphylaxis.**
Warnings	Mild intercurrent illness usually does not present a barrier to vaccination. Vaccines are contraindicated in patients who have had an ✖**anaphylactic reaction to a past dose** or to one of its constituents. Live vaccines are contraindicated in patients with ✖**significant immunosuppression,** and are usually avoided in ▲**pregnancy.**
Important interactions	▲**Immunosuppressive drugs** (including systemic <u>corticosteroids</u>) reduce the immune response to (and therefore effectiveness of) vaccines, and may permit generalised infection with live vaccines.

PRACTICAL PRESCRIBING

Prescription	Vaccines administered as part of the childhood immunisation schedule are in effect 'pre-prescribed' in the **Personal Child Health Record** (their 'Red Book'), either by a GP or an independent nurse prescriber at the 6- to 8-week check (technically this is a 'patient-specific direction'). Vaccines administered outside of this schedule (e.g. for adults) generally need to be prescribed individually. Details are specific for each vaccine product and are provided in the BNF.
Administration	Most vaccines are given by **IM injection.** Usual practice for IM injections applies. In babies, the injection is generally given into the thigh, while in older children and adults the upper arm is used. Where more than one vaccination is required, they should ideally be given in different limbs. The **BCG** (Bacillus Calmette–Guérin) vaccine for tuberculosis is given intradermally, ideally in the region of the insertion of the left deltoid muscle to aid later identification of the scar.
Communication	Explain to the patient, or as appropriate the child's parent, the nature and purpose of the vaccine and the likely side effects. Advise that mild reactions, particularly when they involve fever, can be treated with paracetamol. Parents are free to refuse vaccinations on behalf of their child, but you should offer reasonable encouragement towards acceptance. Explain that there is considerable evidence that benefits of vaccinations far outweigh the risk of side effects.
Monitoring	All individuals who have received a vaccine should be monitored for a few minutes in the surgery because of the very small risk of anaphylactic reaction. Thereafter, the patient or, as appropriate, their parents can monitor and usually self-treat mild reactions. There is usually no need to monitor the serological response to a vaccine, but this may be indicated in a few circumstances (e.g. *hepatitis B vaccination*).
Cost	Assessments of cost effectiveness are integral to the decision to add a vaccine to the childhood vaccination schedule.

Clinical tip—In patients with bleeding disorders (e.g. thrombocytopenia), use deep SC injection in preference to IM injection to avoid causing muscle haematoma.

Valproate

CLINICAL PHARMACOLOGY

Common indications	❶ **Epilepsy,** as a first choice drug for the control of generalised or absence seizures and as a treatment option for focal seizures. ❷ **Bipolar disorder,** for the acute treatment of manic episodes and prophylaxis against recurrence.
Mechanisms of action	The mechanism of action of valproate is incompletely understood. It appears be a weak **inhibitor of neuronal sodium channels,** stabilising resting membrane potentials and reducing neuronal excitability (see Phenytoin). It also **increases** the brain content of γ-aminobutyric acid (GABA), the principal inhibitory neurotransmitter, which regulates neuronal excitability.
Important adverse effects	The most common dose-related adverse events are **gastrointestinal upset** (such as nausea, gastric irritation and diarrhoea), **neurological and psychiatric** effects (including tremor, ataxia and behavioural disturbances), **thrombocytopenia** and transient increase in **liver enzymes.** Hypersensitivity reactions include **hair loss,** with subsequent regrowth being curlier than original hair. Rare, **life-threatening idiosyncratic** adverse effects include severe liver injury, pancreatitis, bone marrow failure and antiepileptic hypersensitivity syndrome (see Carbamazepine).
Warnings	Valproate should be avoided where possible in ✖**women of child-bearing age,** particularly around the time of ✖**conception** and in the ✖**first trimester of pregnancy.** It is the antiepileptic drug associated with the greatest risk of **fetal abnormalities,** including neural tube defects, craniofacial, cardiac and limb abnormalities and developmental delay. It should be avoided in patients with ▲**hepatic impairment** and dose reduction is required in patients with ▲**severe renal impairment.**
Important interactions	Valproate inhibits hepatic cytochrome P450 enzymes, increasing plasma concentration and toxicity of ▲**drugs metabolised by P450 enzymes,** including, for example, warfarin and other antiepileptic drugs. Valproate is itself metabolised by these enzymes. As such, valproate concentration is reduced and risk of seizures may be increased by ▲**cytochrome P450 inducers** (e.g. phenytoin, carbamazepine), and also by carbapenems. Adverse effects are increased by ▲**cytochrome P450 inhibitors** (e.g. macrolides, protease inhibitors) and drugs that **displace it from protein binding sites** (e.g. aspirin). The efficacy of antiepileptic drugs is reduced by ▲**drugs that lower the seizure threshold** (e.g. SSRIs, tricyclic antidepressants, antipsychotics, tramadol).

sodium valproate, valproic acid

PRACTICAL PRESCRIBING

Prescription

Valproate is formulated as a sodium salt, which is prescribed in epilepsy, and as valproic acid, licensed for bipolar disorders. Valproate dose is equivalent in the two formulations, but care is required when switching between them. The usual daily starting dose of valproate is 600 mg for **epilepsy** and 750 mg for **bipolar disorder,** taken in 1–3 divided doses. The dose is increased to a usual daily maximum of 1–2 g.

Administration

Oral valproate is formulated as a bewildering array of normal or enteric-coated tablets, capsules, granules and oral solutions. Some formulations can be crushed (tablets) or mixed with food (granules), whereas modified-release and enteric-coated formulations should be swallowed whole without chewing. It is important to give the patient appropriate instructions for the formulation chosen. **Intravenous valproate** can be used temporarily where oral administration is not possible. It can be given either as a slow IV injection or by infusion.

Communication

Explain that the aim of treatment is to **reduce frequency of seizures.** Warn patients that they may have some indigestion or tummy upset when starting valproate, but that these will settle in a few days and can be reduced by taking **tablets with food.** As the most serious potential adverse effects are unpredictable, patients should seek **urgent medical advice** for unexpected symptoms including lethargy, loss of appetite, vomiting or abdominal pain (may indicate liver poisoning) or bruising, a high temperature or mouth ulcers (may indicate blood abnormalities). For women, discuss **contraception and pregnancy** (see Clinical tip). Advise patients **not to drive** unless they have been seizure-free for 12 months (or have only had seizures when asleep over 3 years). They should not drive for 6 months after changing or stopping treatment.

Monitoring

Monitor **efficacy** by comparing seizure frequency before and after starting treatment or dose adjustment. Monitor **safety** by patient report. Measurement of liver function (including prothrombin time) before and during the first 6 months of treatment may be useful. **Plasma valproate concentrations** (usually 40–100 mg/L) do not correlate well with therapeutic effect. They should therefore only be measured to check for adherence or toxicity.

Cost

Valproate is inexpensive (around £9 for a 100-pack of 500 mg tablets). However, cost increases with complexity of the formulation.

Clinical tip—Women of child-bearing age who need to take valproate should be advised to use effective contraception during treatment. Before conception, review by an epilepsy specialist and folic acid supplementation should be arranged. For unplanned pregnancies during valproate treatment, advise the patient that there is at least a 90% chance of a normal baby. Prenatal monitoring should be offered to detect fetal abnormalities.

Vancomycin

CLINICAL PHARMACOLOGY

Common indications	❶ Treatment of Gram-positive infection, e.g. **endocarditis,** where infection is severe and/or penicillins cannot be used due to resistance (e.g. meticillin-resistant *Staphylococcus aureus* [MRSA]) or allergy. ❷ Treatment of **antibiotic-associated colitis** caused by *Clostridium difficile* infection (usually second-line where metronidazole is ineffective or poorly tolerated).
Mechanisms of action	Vancomycin inhibits growth and cross-linking of peptidoglycan chains, **inhibiting synthesis of the cell wall of Gram-positive bacteria.** It therefore has specific activity against Gram-positive aerobic and anaerobic bacteria and is inactive against most Gram-negative bacteria, which have a different (lipopolysaccharide) cell wall structure. Bacterial resistance to vancomycin is increasingly reported. One mechanism is modification of cell wall structure to prevent vancomycin binding.
Important adverse effects	The most common adverse effect is pain and inflammation of the vein (**thrombophlebitis**) at the infusion site. If vancomycin is infused rapidly, severe adverse reactions can occur. These include anaphylactoid reactions classically described as '**red man syndrome**'. This is characterised by generalised erythema and may be associated with hypotension and bronchospasm. Anaphylactoid reactions are not antigen-mediated (i.e. not true allergy), but are due to non-specific degranulation of mast cells. However, true allergy to vancomycin (**immediate or delayed hypersensitivity**) can also occur. Intravenous vancomycin can cause **nephrotoxicity,** including renal failure and interstitial nephritis, **ototoxicity,** with tinnitus and hearing loss, and **blood disorders,** including neutropenia and thrombocytopenia.
Warnings	Vancomycin treatment requires careful monitoring of plasma drug concentrations and dose adjustment to avoid toxicity. Particular caution including dose reduction should be taken when prescribing for people with ▲**renal impairment** and the ▲**elderly** (increased risk of hearing impairment).
Important interactions	Vancomycin increases the risk of ototoxicity and/or nephrotoxicity when prescribed with aminoglycosides, loop diuretics or ciclosporin (an immunosuppressant drug).

PRACTICAL PRESCRIBING

Prescription	Vancomycin is a large hydrophilic molecule that is very poorly absorbed across lipid membranes. For **systemic infection**, vancomycin must therefore be given intravenously. The initial dosage regimen is determined by renal function and adjusted according to plasma drug concentration (see Monitoring). Antibiotic treatment may be required for several weeks for patients with severe or deep-seated infection, e.g. **endocarditis** or **osteomyelitis.** For *C. difficile* **colitis,** vancomycin must be given orally, typically 125 mg 6-hrly for 10–14 days.
Administration	Oral vancomycin is formulated as capsules, although the powder used for injection can be made up as and taken as an oral solution (cheaper). Intravenous vancomycin must be given by slow infusion (not IV bolus or IM injection) to reduce the risk of anaphylactoid reactions and 'red man syndrome'; 1 g of vancomycin must be diluted in at least 250 mL sodium chloride 0.9% or glucose 5% and infused over at least 60 minutes.
Communication	Explain that the aim of treatment is to get rid of infection and improve symptoms. For oral treatment, encourage the patient to complete the prescribed course. Warn them to **report any ringing in the ears** or change in hearing during treatment, as this is only reversible if treatment is stopped promptly. Vancomycin treatment is relatively uncommon, so patients are unlikely to give a history of prior vancomycin allergy.
Monitoring	Where IV therapy is used, pre-dose (trough) **plasma vancomycin concentrations** should be measured during treatment. Vancomycin dosage should be adjusted to keep plasma concentrations above 10 mg/L to maintain therapeutic effect but below 15 mg/L to minimise toxicity. Check that **infection resolves** by resolution of symptoms, signs (e.g. pyrexia) and blood markers (e.g. falling C-reactive protein and white cell count) as appropriate. Safety monitoring should include daily **renal function** and regular **full blood count monitoring** during prolonged therapy (risk of renal impairment, blood disorders).
Cost	A 14-day course of treatment for *C. difficile* colitis costs around £3 for oral metronidazole and around £200 for vancomycin capsules. Metronidazole is therefore often recommended as first line for suspected *C. difficile* infection.

Clinical tip—Prescription of vancomycin and subsequent monitoring and dosage adjustment is complex. Furthermore, vancomycin treatment is relatively uncommon, so it can be difficult for a junior doctor to gain expertise in this field. Always consult local guidelines and contact microbiology or pharmacy colleagues to ensure vancomycin prescription is done safely and effectively.

Vitamins

CLINICAL PHARMACOLOGY

Common indications	❶ *Thiamine* (vitamin B₁) is used in the treatment and prevention of **Wernicke's encephalopathy** and **Korsakoff's psychosis,** which are manifestations of severe thiamine deficiency. ❷ *Folic acid* (the synthetic form of folate or vitamin B₉) is used in **megaloblastic anaemia** due to folate deficiency, and in the first trimester of pregnancy to reduce the risk of **neural tube defects.** ❸ *Hydroxocobalamin* (a synthetic form of cobalamin or vitamin B₁₂) is used in the treatment of **megaloblastic anaemia** and **subacute combined degeneration of the cord** due to vitamin B₁₂ deficiency. ❹ *Phytomenadione* (the plant form of vitamin K) is recommended for all newborn babies to prevent **vitamin K deficiency bleeding,** and is used to **reverse the anticoagulant effect of <u>warfarin</u>** (prothrombin complex concentrate should also be given in cases of major bleeding).
Mechanisms of action	Vitamins are organic substances required in small amounts for normal metabolic processes. **Vitamin deficiencies** and their associated clinical manifestations may be treated with a pharmaceutical form of the relevant vitamin; the mechanism of action is self-explanatory (see Common indications). In pregnancy and the preconception period, giving folic acid reduces the risk of congenital **neural tube defects.** As it is required for normal cell division, it may work by facilitating cell proliferation involved in neural tube closure, but this is not completely understood. *Phytomenadione* **reverses <u>warfarin</u>** by providing a fresh supply of vitamin K for the synthesis of vitamin K-dependent clotting factors by the liver.
Important adverse effects	When given IV, *phytomenadione* and high-dose *thiamine* may rarely cause **anaphylaxis.** Most other vitamin preparations are relatively non-toxic.
Warnings	In patients with co-existing ▲B₁₂ **and folate deficiency,** you should replace both vitamins simultaneously. This is because replacing *folic acid* alone may be associated with (and perhaps hasten) progression of the neurological manifestations of B₁₂ deficiency. The major concern is the risk of provoking subacute combined degeneration of the cord. *Phytomenadione* is less effective in reversing <u>warfarin</u> in patients with ▲**severe liver disease,** as clotting factors are synthesised in the liver.
Important interactions	As noted above, vitamin K and <u>warfarin</u> have an antagonistic interaction which, initially, is desirable. However, when attempting to restart warfarin after vitamin K has been given, it may result in erratic dosing requirements.

folic acid, thiamine, hydroxocobalamin, phytomenadione

PRACTICAL PRESCRIBING

Prescription	In hospital, patients at high risk of **thiamine deficiency** are best treated initially with *Pabrinex®*, a compound preparation of B and C vitamins. This is prescribed in 'pairs' of ampules. A typical dose for *prophylaxis* in high-risk patients would be 1 pair 12-hrly IV for 3 days. *Treatment* doses are higher. Oral thiamine (e.g. 200 mg daily) is started subsequently. To **prevent neural tube defects,** folic acid 400 micrograms daily should be started before conception ideally, or otherwise at the diagnosis of pregnancy, then continued until week 12. This can be purchased without prescription. Where there is high risk of neural tube defect (e.g. in epilepsy), a higher dose of 5 mg daily is used. This is also the dose used in **folate deficiency anaemia. In vitamin B$_{12}$ deficiency,** hydroxocobalamin is given by IM injection. Oral cyanocobalamin is an alternative, but as the problem is usually with B$_{12}$ absorption, it is best avoided. To prevent **vitamin K deficiency bleeding** in neonates, phytomenadione 1 mg IM is given as a single dose (lower doses in preterm neonates). To treat an excessively high international normalised ratio (INR) in **warfarin therapy,** it is best to give a low dose of phytomenadione (e.g. 1 mg orally or IV). In cases of major bleeding, 10 mg IV is given. Consult a local protocol or the BNF for further guidance.
Administration	Each carton of *Pabrinex®* contains 2 ampules labelled No 1 and No 2. The contents of both ampules are added to a small bag (50–100 mL) of 0.9% sodium chloride or 5% glucose, mixed, and infused over 30 minutes. *Phytomenadione*, when given IV, should always be injected very slowly.
Communication	It is always worth raising the issue of folic acid supplementation in a consultation with a woman of child-bearing age, due to the benefits of starting this in the preconception period.
Monitoring	Treatment of **thiamine deficiency** is monitored clinically. Treatment of **folate** and **B$_{12}$ deficiency** are monitored clinically and with the full blood count. The effect of **phytomenadione** on the INR becomes evident 12–24 hours after administration. No monitoring is required after prophylactic use in neonates.
Cost	Most vitamin preparations are inexpensive.

Clinical tip—In patients taking warfarin, a high INR with no bleeding may be corrected with a small oral dose of vitamin K (e.g. 0.5–1 mg). This is preferred to higher doses which may make subsequent dosing erratic. The usual oral formulation of vitamin K stocked on adult wards is menadiol phosphate, but this only comes in 10 mg tablets. An alternative, therefore, is to use phytomenadione solution intended for IV administration but give it orally. The easiest way to do this is to draw 1 mL of the 10 mg/mL solution into a syringe, add 9 mL of water, then give 1 mL (1 mg) of the resultant solution.

Warfarin

CLINICAL PHARMACOLOGY

Common indications	❶ To prevent clot extension and recurrence in **deep vein thrombosis** and **pulmonary embolism** (collectively, venous thromboembolism [VTE]). ❷ To prevent embolic complications (e.g. stroke) in **atrial fibrillation.** ❸ To prevent embolic complications (e.g. stroke) after **heart valve replacement.** Treatment is short term after tissue valve replacement and lifelong for mechanical valve replacement. Warfarin is not used to prevent *arterial thrombosis* (e.g. myocardial infarction, thrombotic stroke). As this is driven by platelet aggregation, it is prevented by antiplatelet agents, such as aspirin and clopidogrel.
Mechanisms of action	Warfarin inhibits hepatic production of vitamin K-dependent coagulation factors and cofactors. Vitamin K must be in its reduced form for synthesis of coagulation factors. It is then oxidised during the synthetic process. An enzyme called vitamin K epoxide reductase reactivates oxidised vitamin K. Warfarin **inhibits vitamin K epoxide reductase, preventing** reactivation of vitamin K and **coagulation factor synthesis.**
Important adverse effects	The main adverse effect of warfarin is **bleeding.** A slight excess of warfarin increases the risk of bleeding from existing abnormalities such as peptic ulcers or following minor trauma (e.g. intracerebral haemorrhage after minor head injury). A large excess of warfarin can trigger spontaneous haemorrhage such epistaxis (nose bleed) or retroperitoneal haemorrhage.
Warnings	As there is a fine line between thrombosis and haemorrhage in patients taking warfarin, potential risks and benefits must be carefully balanced. Warfarin is contraindicated in patients at ✖**immediate risk of haemorrhage,** including after trauma and in patients requiring surgery. Patients with ▲**liver disease** who are less able to metabolise the drug are at risk of over-anticoagulation/bleeding. In ✖**pregnancy,** warfarin should not be used in the first trimester as it causes fetal malformations, including cardiac and cranial abnormalities. It should not be used towards term, when it may cause maternal haemorrhage at delivery.
Important interactions	The plasma concentration of warfarin required to prevent clotting is very close to the concentration that causes bleeding (**low therapeutic index**). Small changes in hepatic warfarin metabolism by cytochrome P450 enzymes can cause clinically significant changes in anticoagulation. ▲**Cytochrome P450 inhibitors** (e.g. fluconazole, macrolides, protease inhibitors) decrease warfarin metabolism and increase bleeding risk. ▲**Cytochrome P450 inducers** (e.g. phenytoin, carbamazepine, rifampicin) increase warfarin metabolism and risk of clots. Many antibiotics can increase anticoagulation in patients on warfarin by killing gut flora which synthesise vitamin K.

PRACTICAL PRESCRIBING

Prescription	Warfarin is taken orally once a day. The dose is 5–10 mg on day 1, with the lower dose used for patients who are elderly, lighter or at increased bleeding risk (e.g. due to interacting medicines). Subsequent doses are guided by the **international normalised ratio** (INR). After starting warfarin, it takes several days for full anticoagulation to be achieved. Patients needing immediate anticoagulation usually start both heparin (fast onset of action) and warfarin. Heparin is withdrawn when full anticoagulation with warfarin is achieved. A single episode of VTE is treated with warfarin for 3–6 months. Lifelong warfarin may be required for recurrent VTE or cardiac disease. However, treatment may be stopped if new bleeding risks exceed potential benefits.
Administration	Traditionally, warfarin is taken each day at around 18:00 hours for consistent effects on the INR taken the following morning. This may also help patients remember when to take it (around tea time). The comedian Paul O'Grady, who takes the drug, has been known to remind his afternoon radio listeners that 'it's time for our warfarin!'
Communication	Advise patients that warfarin treatment is a balance between benefits (preventing clots) and risks (bleeding). It is important for patients to understand how food, alcohol and other drugs can affect warfarin treatment. Patients receive an **anticoagulant book ('Yellow Book')**, which acts as an alert to their warfarin therapy and is used to record warfarin doses, blood test results, treatment indication and duration.
Monitoring	The INR is the prothrombin time of a person on warfarin divided by that of a non-warfarinised 'control'. **INR target values** vary by indication for warfarin. For example, in atrial fibrillation and VTE the target range is usually 2.0–3.0. INR is measured daily in hospital inpatients and every few days in outpatients commencing warfarin. Once a stable dose of warfarin has been established, INR measurement is less frequent.
Cost	Warfarin costs about £1/month, but associated monitoring costs add to this. **Novel oral anticoagulants** (NOACs, e.g. dabigatran, rivaroxaban) have similar efficacy to warfarin, slightly better safety profiles and require less intensive monitoring. However, at £60–£70/month their cost is likely to present barriers as the NHS seeks to adopt them.

Clinical tip—Dosing warfarin can be a challenge. Follow local guidelines if possible, and if in doubt seek advice from the anticoagulation service. Changes in INR lag behind changes in the warfarin dose. Look back over the last 48–72 hours to see what doses have led to the current INR. Avoid large dose swings wherever possible.

Z-drugs

CLINICAL PHARMACOLOGY

Common indications	❶ Short-term treatment of **insomnia** which is debilitating or distressing.
Mechanisms of action	The 'Z-drugs' have a similar mechanism of action to <u>benzodiazepines</u>, although they are chemically quite distinct. Their target is the γ-aminobutyric acid type A (GABA$_A$) receptor. The GABA$_A$ receptor is a chloride channel that opens in response to binding by GABA, the main inhibitory neurotransmitter in the brain. Opening the channel allows chloride to flow into the cell, making the cell more resistant to depolarisation. Like benzodiazepines, **Z-drugs facilitate and enhance binding of GABA to the GABA$_A$ receptor.** This has a widespread depressant effect on synaptic transmission. The clinical manifestations of this include reduced anxiety, sleepiness, and sedation. Note that they are not useful anticonvulsants, as they can only be taken orally. In general, Z-drugs have a shorter duration of action than benzodiazepines.
Important adverse effects	All Z-drugs can cause **daytime sleepiness,** which may affect ability to drive or perform complex tasks the day after taking the medication. **Rebound insomnia** may occur when the drugs are stopped. Other **central nervous system effects** include headache, confusion, nightmares and (rarely) amnesia. As Z-drugs are chemically distinct from each other, their adverse effects differ. *Zopiclone* can cause **taste disturbance,** whereas *zolpidem* more commonly causes **gastrointestinal upset.** Prolonged used of Z-drugs beyond 4 weeks can lead to **dependence,** with **withdrawal symptoms** on stopping, including headaches, muscle pains and anxiety. In overdose, Z-drugs cause **drowsiness, coma and respiratory depression.**
Warnings	Z-drugs should be used with caution in the ▲**elderly,** who are often more sensitive to drugs with central nervous system effects. They should not be prescribed for patients with ✖**obstructive sleep apnoea** or those with ✖**respiratory muscle weakness** or **respiratory depression,** in whom they may worsen respiratory failure during sleep.
Important interactions	Z-drugs enhance the sedative effects of alcohol, <u>antihistamines</u> and benzodiazepines. They enhance the hypotensive effect of antihypertensive medications. As Z-drugs are metabolised by cytochrome P450 enzymes, ▲**P450 inhibitors** (e.g. <u>macrolides</u>) can enhance sedation, whereas **P450 inducers** (e.g. <u>phenytoin</u>, rifampicin) can impair sedation.

PRACTICAL PRESCRIBING

Prescription	Hypnotics, such as Z-drugs, should only be prescribed for short-term use in the treatment of insomnia, for a maximum of 4 weeks. Typical doses are zopiclone 7.5 mg or zolpidem 10 mg, to be taken at bedtime. Starting doses should be halved for elderly patients.
Administration	The Z-drugs are only available for oral administration as tablets or capsules.
Communication	When treating insomnia, explain to patients that 'sleeping tablets' should only be used as a **short-term measure** to help them get over a bad patch. Discuss reasons why they are not sleeping and offer advice on 'sleep hygiene'. Advise them to take 'sleeping tablets' **only when really needed,** as the body can get used to them if taken regularly. Warn them that the maximum time they should use the tablets for is **4 weeks,** as if used for longer they may become dependent on them and may feel unwell when they stop taking them. Warn them **not to drive or operate complex or heavy machinery** after taking the drug and explain that sometimes sleepiness may persist the following day.
Monitoring	Efficacy and safety are monitored clinically.
Cost	Both zopiclone and zolpidem are available in non-proprietary preparations and are relatively inexpensive.

Clinical tip—The routine prescription of hypnotics, such as Z-drugs, is not recommended for the treatment of insomnia because of the potential for tolerance and dependence and because it does not address the underlying cause of insomnia. However, hypnotics are very useful as short-term treatment in *specific* circumstances, e.g. for an anxious patient wishing to get a good night's sleep prior to surgery or for recently bereaved people for whom insomnia is a significant problem.

5α-reductase inhibitors

CLINICAL PHARMACOLOGY

Common indications	**❶ In benign prostatic hyperplasia,** 5α-reductase inhibitors are a second-line medical treatment after <u>α-blockers</u>. They improve lower urinary tract symptoms, such as difficulty passing urine, urinary retention and poor urinary flow, and reduce the need for prostate-related surgery.
Mechanisms of action	5α-reductase inhibitors reduce the size of the prostate gland. They do this by **inhibiting** the intracellular enzyme **5α-reductase,** which converts testosterone to its more active metabolite dihydrotestosterone. As dihydrotestosterone stimulates prostatic growth, inhibition of its production by 5α-reductase inhibitors reduces prostatic enlargement and improves urinary flow. However, it can take several months for this effect to become evident clinically. For this reason, an <u>α-blocker</u> is usually preferred for initial therapy, with a 5α-reductase inhibitor added if the response is poor or if the prostate is particularly bulky.
Important adverse effects	The most common adverse effects of 5α-reductase inhibitors relate to their anti-androgen action. These include **impotence** and **reduced libido,** which are usually transient, and breast tenderness and enlargement (**gynaecomastia**), which can affect patient adherence to treatment. An additional effect of androgen inhibition is **hair growth,** which can be exploited to advantage in treatment of male-pattern baldness. **Breast cancer** has been reported in men taking finasteride.
Warnings	Exposure of a male foetus to 5α-reductase inhibitors may cause abnormal development of the external genitalia. It is therefore important that ✖**pregnant women** do not take these drugs and are not exposed to them, e.g. by handling broken or damaged tablets or through semen during unprotected intercourse with a man taking these drugs.
Important interactions	There are no clinically important drug interactions.

PRACTICAL PRESCRIBING

Prescription	Finasteride is taken orally. The usual dose for the treatment of benign prostatic hypertrophy is 5 mg daily.
Administration	Women of child-bearing potential should avoid handling crushed or broken tablets.
Communication	Explain to the patient that the reason he is having difficulty passing urine is because his prostate has grown and is squashing the tube coming out of the bladder. Tell him that finasteride treatment will **make his prostate shrink,** which will open up the tube and make it **easier to pass urine.** However, it may take **up to 6 months** before symptoms improve. Warn him of the **main side effects,** particularly that he may feel less keen to have sex and may be less able to get or keep an erection. It is important to point out that these problems will only last for a short while and normal function should return as treatment continues. Explain that he may also notice some tenderness or growth in the tissue underneath his nipples. If this occurs he should see his doctor. Explain these changes are usually harmless, however very rarely men can get breast cancer and this is slightly more likely on this drug. Encourage the patient to return if he is having a lot of trouble with side effects, as other treatments for his enlarged prostate could be considered. If the patient has a partner who is or could become pregnant, advise him to use a condom during intercourse to protect the baby from the effects of the drug.
Monitoring	Schedule a follow-up appointment in 3–6 months to review changes in lower urinary tract symptoms and the development of adverse effects. Continue check-ups every 6–12 months while treatment continues.
Cost	Finasteride is available in non-proprietary form and is inexpensive.

Clinical tip—Finasteride is a good example of the importance of **post-marketing surveillance.** In clinical trials, relatively few carefully selected patients (hundreds to thousands) are exposed to a drug and common adverse effects are identified. After marketing, many more patients (thousands to millions) with less stringent selection criteria are exposed to the drug and less common adverse effects may emerge. In the UK, suspected adverse effects of medicines should be reported to the Medicines and Healthcare Products Regulatory Agency (**MHRA**) by health professionals or the public using the **Yellow Card scheme.** For finasteride, there were reports of breast cancer in clinical trials, but these were not statistically associated with drug use. Continued reports of breast cancer during post-marketing surveillance led to a review of its safety and changes in the information given to patients about breast cancer risk.

Fluids

Colloids (plasma substitutes)

CLINICAL PHARMACOLOGY

Common indications	❶ Colloids are used to **expand circulating volume** in states of **circulatory compromise** (including **shock**). However, we prefer compound sodium lactate or sodium chloride 0.9% for this indication. ❷ In **cirrhotic liver disease,** albumin is used to prevent effective hypovolaemia in **large-volume paracentesis** (ascitic fluid drainage).
Mechanisms of action	In relation to fluid therapy, a colloid is a solution containing a **large, osmotically active molecule,** such as albumin or modified gelatin. In principle, the large molecules cannot readily diffuse out of vessels, and their osmotic effect 'holds' the infused fluid in the plasma. For example, under experimental conditions, 70–80% of a gelatin-based fluid remains in the plasma. Their effect in **expanding circulating volume** is therefore potentially greater than that of a crystalloid (e.g. sodium chloride), of which around 20% remains in the plasma after distribution. In practice, however, most patients requiring volume expansion (e.g. in severe sepsis) have relatively 'leaky' capillaries, and it is likely that some of the gelatin is lost into the interstitium. There is no convincing evidence that the use of colloids rather than crystalloids improves clinical outcomes, and trials using starch-based colloids have demonstrated harm. We therefore favour crystalloids for this indication. **Large-volume paracentesis** (generally defined as >5 L) in **cirrhotic liver disease** can produce adverse haemodynamic effects. It is customary to administer human albumin solution (HAS) in an attempt to prevent this, although the evidence supporting this practice is much debated.
Important adverse effects	Excessive administration of colloid fluids may cause a fall in cardiac output and precipitate **cardiac failure** by increasing left ventricular filling beyond the point of maximal contractility on the Starling curve. Most colloids contain a significant amount of sodium (e.g. 154 mmol/L in the case of Gelofusine®) and this may produce **oedema.** Gelatins may cause **hypersensitivity reactions,** including anaphylaxis – another reason to prefer crystalloids, which are non-allergenic.
Warnings	Fluid volume should be reduced in patients with ▲**heart failure,** due to the risk of worsening myocardial contractility. In ▲**renal impairment,** it is vital to monitor fluid balance closely to avoid overload.
Important interactions	There are no clinically important interactions.

PRACTICAL PRESCRIBING

Prescription	Colloids are prescribed in the 'infusions' section of the drug chart. Synthetic colloids are generally prescribed by brand name. You need to specify the volume to be infused and the rate at which it is to be given. The rate may be described either in mL per hour or as the intended duration for infusion of the total volume. For example, if deemed appropriate to use a colloid in **circulatory compromise** or **shock,** you might prescribe 250 mL of Gelofusine® to be given over 10 minutes (equivalent to 1500 mL/hr). In the context of **large-volume paracentesis,** you should consult with specialist colleagues regarding the need for albumin. A common regimen is to give 100 mL of HAS 20% for every 2 L of ascitic fluid drained.
Administration	Infusions may be administered simply through a giving set, in which case the flow is controlled with a roller valve and the rate estimated from the number of drips per minute. Alternatively, and preferably, an infusion pump can be used to control the rate more precisely. A pressure bag can be applied to help infuse the fluid more quickly.
Communication	Explain that you advise treatment with fluid through a drip in order to (for example) improve their blood pressure. Ask the patient to report any irritation, swelling or wetness around the cannula site, as this may indicate that the cannula is no longer functioning correctly.
Monitoring	Patients requiring expansion of circulating volume are sick and require close monitoring. It is vital to assess haemodynamic status (e.g. pulse, blood pressure, jugular venous pressure, capillary refill time, urine output) before and after infusion as a guide to further therapy. Similarly, close monitoring is required in the context of large-volume paracentesis to detect adverse haemodynamic consequences, whether due to ascitic fluid drainage or albumin administration.
Cost	Colloid solutions are considerably more expensive than crystalloids.

Clinical tip—In managing a severely ill patient requiring large-volume fluid therapy, it is a good idea to use warmed fluids if possible, to avoid causing hypothermia. A fluid-warming cabinet (hopefully containing some warm bags of fluid) can usually be found in the operating department, emergency department, or intensive care unit.

Compound sodium lactate (Hartmann's solution)

CLINICAL PHARMACOLOGY

Common indications	❶ To **provide sodium and water intravenously** in patients unable to take enough orally. ❷ To **expand circulating volume** in states of **circulatory compromise** (including **shock**). This may be done as a 'fluid challenge', where a selected volume of fluid (e.g. 500 mL) is infused rapidly. <u>Sodium chloride 0.9%</u> and <u>colloids</u> are alternatives.
Mechanisms of action	Compound sodium lactate (more commonly known by its eponymous name, Hartmann's solution) is a 'balanced salt solution'. Its constituents are designed to mimic serum, at least in terms of electrolytes. One litre contains Na^+ 131 mmol, Cl^- 111 mmol, K^+ 5 mmol, Ca^{2+} 2 mmol, and lactate 29 mmol. In the presence of adequate liver function, the lactate is metabolised to pyruvate and then either to glucose or carbon dioxide and water, with the release of bicarbonate in both cases. The sodium content means it may be used to provide sodium and water intravenously, and also for the expansion of circulating volume (see <u>Sodium chloride</u>).
Important adverse effects	Excessive administration of compound sodium lactate can cause a fall in cardiac output and severe **heart failure** by increasing left ventricular filling beyond the point of maximal contractility on the Starling curve. **Oedema** may be caused by providing sodium more rapidly than the patient can excrete it. This is especially relevant in patients who have received multiple fluid challenges, since about 80% of the administered volume will have been 'lost' into tissue fluid. The main advantage of compound sodium lactate over <u>sodium chloride 0.9%</u> is its lower chloride content. It is thus less likely to cause hyperchloraemic acidosis.
Warnings	Fluid challenge volume should be reduced in patients with ▲**heart failure,** due to the risk of worsening myocardial contractility. In ▲**renal impairment,** it is vital to monitor fluid balance closely to avoid overload. Moreover, although the potassium content is low, you should monitor the serum potassium concentration if it is used in this context. Compound sodium lactate is best avoided in ▲**severe liver disease** because there may not be sufficient capacity to metabolise lactate.
Important interactions	There are no clinically important interactions.

compound sodium lactate (Hartmann's solution)

PRACTICAL PRESCRIBING

Prescription	Compound sodium lactate is prescribed in the 'infusions' section of the drug chart. You need to specify the volume to be infused and the rate at which it is to be given. The rate may be described either in mL per hour or as the intended duration for infusion of the total volume. For example, in **providing sodium intravenously,** you might prescribe 500 mL of compound sodium lactate for administration over 4 hours (equivalent to 125 mL/hr). This would provide 66 mmol of sodium, covering their daily 'maintenance' requirement. You would probably also prescribe glucose 5% to provide their remaining water requirement (about 2 L/day). To **expand circulating volume,** you might prescribe 500 mL of compound sodium lactate to be given over 15 minutes (equivalent to 2000 mL/hr).
Administration	Infusions may be administered simply through a giving set, in which case the flow is controlled with a roller valve and the rate estimated from the number of drips per minute. Alternatively, and preferably, an infusion pump can be used to control the rate more precisely.
Communication	Explain that you are offering treatment with a drip because (for example) they are unable to take enough fluid by mouth. As appropriate, encourage the patient to drink more, explaining that this is much better than giving fluid artificially. Ask the patient to report any irritation, swelling or wetness around the cannula site, as this may indicate that the cannula is no longer functioning correctly.
Monitoring	In any patient receiving fluid infusions, fluid balance should be monitored and recorded (see Glucose). In the context of **circulatory compromise,** it is vital to assess haemodynamic status (e.g. pulse, blood pressure, jugular venous pressure, capillary refill time, urine output) before and after infusion as a guide to further therapy.
Cost	Compound sodium lactate solutions are inexpensive. However, associated costs (including infusion equipment, consumables, staff time and treatment of complications) may be considerable.

Clinical tip—By virtue of its slightly lower sodium content and its substantially lower chloride content, compound sodium lactate is probably a better fluid than sodium chloride 0.9% in most circumstances. There is a lot to be said for using it as your 'standard' sodium-based fluid. The main caveats are that it should be avoided in severe liver and renal disease (due to its lactate and potassium content, respectively), and that it offers less flexibility in terms of potassium replacement (as this is fixed at 5 mmol/L, whereas sodium chloride and glucose are routinely available in combination with potassium chloride in concentrations of 20 and 40 mmol/L).

Glucose (dextrose)

CLINICAL PHARMACOLOGY

Common indications	❶ Glucose 5% is used to **provide water intravenously** in patients unable to take enough orally. ❷ Glucose 10%, 20% and 50% are used to treat **hypoglycaemia** when this is severe or cannot be treated orally. Glucagon is an alternative. ❸ Glucose 10%, 20% and 50% are used with <u>insulin</u> to treat **hyperkalaemia.** <u>Calcium gluconate</u> may also be given in this setting. ❹ Glucose 5% is used for **reconstitution and dilution of drugs** intended for administration by injection or infusion. <u>Sodium chloride 0.9%</u> and sterile water are alternatives.
Mechanisms of action	Glucose ($C_6H_{12}O_6$) is a monosaccharide that is the principal source of energy for cellular metabolism. It exists in several isomeric configurations, of which D-glucose (dextrose) is the one used in nature. When given in a 5% solution, glucose is administered simply **as a means of providing water intravenously** (its calorific content is negligible). The glucose makes the solution initially isotonic and prevents it from inducing osmolysis. Glucose is rapidly taken up by cells and metabolised, leaving 'free' (hypotonic) water that diffuses throughout all body water compartments. As only about 7% of the administered volume remains in the intravascular space (since the intravascular compartment is about 7% of total body water), glucose is not a suitable fluid for expanding circulating volume. Higher-concentration glucose solutions are used to treat **hypoglycaemia;** the mechanism for this is self-explanatory. In **hyperkalaemia,** <u>insulin</u> (usually Actrapid®) is given to stimulate Na⁺/K⁺-ATPase and shift potassium into cells. Glucose is given simply to prevent hypoglycaemia.
Important adverse effects	**Glucose 50% is highly irritant to veins** and may cause local pain, phlebitis and thrombosis. For this reason, its use is now discouraged, unless it can be given via a central line. Glucose 20% is also irritant, but less so. **Hyperglycaemia** will occur if glucose administration exceeds its utilisation (which is most likely in patients with diabetes mellitus).
Warnings	In patients at risk of ▲**thiamine deficiency,** giving IV glucose can cause **Wernicke's encephalopathy.** If IV glucose treatment is needed, <u>thiamine</u> (as Pabrinex®) must also be given. In ▲**renal failure,** close monitoring of fluid balance is essential to avoid overload. Administering a significant volume of hypotonic fluid to a patient with ▲**hyponatraemia** (or more susceptible to its effects, e.g. ▲**children**) may precipitate hyponatraemic encephalopathy.
Important interactions	Glucose and <u>insulin</u> have antagonistic effects. Concurrent administration may nevertheless be appropriate, as in intravenous insulin infusions, for example. However, the rate of glucose infusion should ideally be kept constant unless treatment for hypoglycaemia is required.

glucose 5%, glucose 10%, glucose 20%, glucose 50%

PRACTICAL PRESCRIBING

Prescription	Glucose 5% is generally prescribed in the 'infusions' section of the drug chart. Although the term 'dextrose' is biologically correct, 'glucose' is the approved name for prescriptions. You need to specify the volume to be infused and the rate at which it is to be given. The rate may be described either in mL per hour or as the intended duration for infusion of the total volume. For example, in **providing water intravenously,** you might prescribe 1 L of glucose 5% for administration over 10 hours (equivalent to 100 mL/hr). This might be part of a daily regimen comprised of, for example, 2 L of 5% glucose and 500 mL of <u>sodium chloride 0.9%</u>, covering the typical 'maintenance' water and sodium requirements in adults. For treatment of **hypoglycaemia,** you might prescribe 100 mL of glucose 10% for infusion over 1–2 minutes. In **hyperkalaemia,** a prescription for 100 mL of glucose 20% with <u>Actrapid</u>® 10 units, to be given over 30 minutes, would be reasonable. For **reconstitution and dilution of drugs,** refer to the BNF or a local policy for details of which fluid to use and what volume to prescribe.
Administration	Infusions may be administered simply through a giving set, in which case the flow is controlled with a roller valve, and the rate estimated from the number of drips per minute. Alternatively, and preferably, an infusion pump can be used to control the rate more precisely.
Communication	For patients receiving IV fluid replacement, explain (as appropriate) that they should still try to take fluid by mouth, as this is much better than providing it artificially. Patients with severe hypoglycaemia may be uncooperative, but should be strongly encouraged to accept treatment before unconsciousness supervenes.
Monitoring	When using glucose to **provide water intravenously,** fluid balance should be monitored. This consists of measuring fluid input (including oral intake and infusions) and output (urine output and additional losses, e.g. from surgical drains), and calculating the net fluid balance (input minus output) for each 24 hour period. In the treatment of **hypoglycaemia** and **hyperkalaemia,** the plasma glucose and serum potassium concentrations should be monitored closely.
Cost	Glucose solutions are inexpensive. However, associated costs (including infusion equipment, consumables, staff time and treatment of complications) may be considerable.

Clinical tip—In a patient that requires both a red cell transfusion and IV glucose, do not allow these to mix (i.e. in the infusion set), as this may cause agglomeration of cells. If appropriate, administer them sequentially rather than concurrently. Alternatively, give them through different cannulas.

Potassium, intravenous

CLINICAL PHARMACOLOGY

Common indications	❶ For **prevention of potassium depletion** in patients unable to take adequate amounts orally. ❷ For **treatment of established potassium depletion and hypokalaemia** that is severe (<2.5 mmol/L), symptomatic, or causing arrhythmias.
Mechanisms of action	The normal potassium requirement to **prevent potassium depletion** is about 1 mmol/kg/day in adults. In patients unable to tolerate dietary intake, who are instead receiving their sodium and water requirement by IV infusion, potassium must also be provided intravenously. **Established potassium depletion and hypokalaemia** may be caused, for example, by diarrhoea, vomiting, or secondary hyperaldosteronism. In severe cases, hypokalaemia may result in arrhythmias (which may be life-threatening), muscle weakness and (in extreme cases) paralysis. IV potassium repletion in these scenarios may be life-saving. For the best effect, IV potassium is given with <u>sodium chloride</u> rather than <u>glucose</u>. This is because the negatively charged chloride ions promote retention of K^+ in the serum for longer, whereas glucose may promote insulin release with resultant stimulation of Na^+/K^+-ATPase, shifting potassium into cells.
Important adverse effects	The major risk of IV potassium infusion is overcorrection leading to **hyperkalaemia** and a resultant risk of **arrhythmias.** Close monitoring is essential to avoid this. Potassium-containing solutions are **irritant to veins** if infused rapidly or in too high concentration. For this reason, the infusion rate in a peripheral vein should generally not exceed 20 mmol/hr.
Warnings	It is unnecessary and potentially dangerous to prescribe potassium for the prevention of potassium depletion in patients with ▲**renal impairment** or ▲**oliguria,** as they have minimal potassium losses and are very susceptible to hyperkalaemia. In the unusual situation in which potassium depletion and hypokalaemia develop in these settings, extreme caution should be exercised in their treatment.
Important interactions	Intravenous potassium has an additive effect with other ▲**potassium-elevating drugs,** including <u>oral potassium</u> supplements, <u>aldosterone antagonists</u>, <u>potassium-sparing diuretics</u>, <u>ACE inhibitors</u> and <u>angiotensin-receptor blockers</u>.

potassium chloride (as a constituent of IV fluid preparations)

PRACTICAL PRESCRIBING

Prescription	Potassium chloride is not available as a 'stand-alone' solution on general wards. Instead, it is prescribed as an ingredient in <u>sodium chloride</u> and <u>glucose</u> solutions, in concentrations of 20 or 40 mmol/L, and in <u>compound sodium lactate</u> at a fixed concentration of 5 mmol/L. Although potassium chloride is added at the manufacturing stage, it is still generally easiest to describe potassium chloride as an 'additive' on the prescription (this is not necessary for compound sodium lactate). Thus, you might write a prescription for 1 L of sodium chloride 0.9% and then, in the additives box, prescribe 'potassium 20 mmol'. The nurse would then select a ready-made bag of sodium chloride 0.9% with potassium chloride 0.15%. The potassium content of 20 mmol is usually printed on the bag in red ink.
Administration	For routine use in prevention of potassium depletion, there are no special considerations for the administration of potassium other than those for fluid replacement in general. In the treatment of established potassium depletion and hypokalaemia, when more rapid infusion rates are likely to be required, IV potassium should ideally be given into a large vein under close monitoring.
Communication	In the context of established potassium depletion and hypokalaemia, advise patients that they have a low level of potassium in their blood, and without treatment this could upset their heart rhythm. You are therefore offering treatment with potassium via a drip. You will need to monitor them closely during this, including with blood tests. This is to ensure the low potassium level is corrected, but not overcorrected, because this too can be risky.
Monitoring	When prescribing potassium for patients unable to take adequate amounts orally, it is prudent to check the serum potassium concentration intermittently. If the patient has renal impairment or oliguria, this should be done every day. When treating established potassium depletion and hypokalaemia, the cardiac rhythm and serum potassium concentration should be monitored closely.
Cost	Cost is not a factor in prescribing decisions for hypokalaemia.

Clinical tip—Hypokalaemia is often associated with hypomagnesaemia. When it is, it may be difficult to correct unless magnesium is also replaced. Always check the magnesium level and prescribe magnesium replacement if necessary (seek advice on how to do this).

Sodium chloride

CLINICAL PHARMACOLOGY

Common indications	❶ Sodium chloride 0.9% and 0.45% are used to **provide sodium and water intravenously** in patients unable to take enough orally. ❷ Sodium chloride 0.9% is used to **expand circulating volume** in states of **circulatory compromise** (including **shock**). Compound sodium lactate and colloids are alternatives. ❸ Sodium chloride 0.9% is used for **reconstitution and dilution of drugs** intended for administration by injection or infusion. Glucose solutions and sterile water are alternatives.
Mechanisms of action	Extracellular fluid (ECF) comprises intravascular and interstitial fluid. Extracellular sodium concentrations are maintained at around 140 mmol/L by Na^+/K^+-ATPase, which pumps sodium out of cells in exchange for potassium. As the main cation in extracellular fluid, sodium is the principal determinant of its osmolality. As the body seeks to keep osmolality constant, an increase in body sodium results in an increase in extracellular water volume. Administration of sodium chloride therefore **expands ECF volume** (until the excess sodium is excreted). The amount by which it expands depends on the sodium concentration of the fluid relative to the ECF. Sodium chloride 0.9% contains 154 mmol/L sodium and is therefore *roughly* isotonic with ECF. This means that ECF expands by approximately the same amount as the volume of sodium chloride 0.9% administered. About 20% of this remains in the intravascular space to **expand circulating volume.** Sodium chloride 0.9% and 0.45% are also used to **provide sodium and water intravenously.** The normal sodium requirement for adults is about 1 mmol/kg/day. This may be increased in disease states, for example due to diarrhoea.
Important adverse effects	Excessive administration of sodium chloride can cause a fall in cardiac output and precipitate **heart failure** by increasing left ventricular filling beyond the point of maximal contractility on the Starling curve. **Oedema** may be caused by providing sodium more rapidly than the patient can excrete it. This is especially relevant in patients who have received large amounts of fluid for circulatory compromise, since about 80% of the administered volume will have been 'lost' into interstitial fluid. Also, sodium chloride 0.9% contains 154 mmol/L of chloride, compared with about 100 mmol/L in ECF. The **hyperchloraemia** that may result from large-volume infusion can generate **acidosis,** due to increased urinary losses of bicarbonate.
Warnings	Fluid challenge volume should be reduced in patients with ▲**heart failure,** due to the risk of worsening cardiac contractility. In ▲**renal impairment,** it is vital to monitor fluid balance closely to avoid overload.
Important interactions	There are no clinically important interactions.

sodium chloride 0.9%, sodium chloride 0.45%

PRACTICAL PRESCRIBING

Prescription	Sodium chloride is generally prescribed in the 'infusions' section of the drug chart. Write 'sodium chloride 0.9%' rather than 'normal saline', since the latter is misleading and is not printed on product labelling. You need to specify the volume to be infused and the rate at which it is to be given. The rate may be described either in mL per hour, or as the intended duration for infusion of the total volume. For example, when **providing sodium intravenously,** you might prescribe 500 mL of sodium chloride 0.9% for administration over 4 hours (equivalent to 125 mL/hr). This would provide 77 mmol of sodium, covering their daily 'maintenance' requirement. You would probably also prescribe <u>glucose 5%</u> to provide their remaining water requirement (about 2 L/day). To **expand circulating volume,** you might prescribe 500 mL of sodium chloride 0.9% to be given over 15 minutes (equivalent to 2000 mL/hr). For **reconstitution and dilution of drugs,** refer to the BNF or a local policy for details of which fluid to use and what volume to prescribe.
Administration	Infusions may be administered simply through a giving set, in which case the flow is controlled with a roller valve, and the rate estimated from the number of drips per minute. Alternatively, and preferably, an infusion pump can be used to control the rate more precisely.
Communication	Explain that you are offering treatment with a drip because (for example) they are unable to take enough fluid by mouth. As appropriate, encourage the patient to drink more, explaining that this is much better than giving fluid artificially. Ask the patient to report any irritation, swelling or wetness around the cannula, as this may indicate that the cannula is no longer functioning correctly.
Monitoring	In any patient receiving fluid infusions, fluid balance should be monitored and recorded (see <u>Glucose</u>). In the context of **circulatory compromise,** it is vital to assess haemodynamic status (e.g. pulse, blood pressure, jugular venous pressure, capillary refill time, urine output) before and after infusion as a guide to further therapy.
Cost	Sodium chloride itself is inexpensive. However, associated costs (including infusion equipment, consumables, staff time and treatment of complications) may be considerable.

Clinical tip—When administering a fluid to **expand circulating volume,** consider using a blood product giving set. This permits a higher flow rate than a standard giving set.

Self-assessment and knowledge integration

Tags used to identify focus areas:

Systems

CVS	Cardiovascular system
RS	Respiratory system
NS	Nervous system
GIS	Gastrointestinal system
Renal/GU	Renal/genitourinary tracts
MSK	Musculoskeletal system
Blood	Blood
Infection	Infection
Skin	Skin
Poisoning	Poisoning
Fluids	Fluids

Topics

Indications	Common indications
Mechanisms	Mechanisms of action
AEs	Important adverse effects
Warnings	Warnings
Interactions	Important interactions
Prescription	Prescription
Admin	Administration
Comm	Communication
Monitoring	Monitoring

1. A 52-year-old man sees his GP with episodic chest pain that occurs on exertion. His GP makes a diagnosis of stable angina.

What treatment would be most likely to prevent further chest pain?

A   Aspirin
B   Bisoprolol
C   Glyceryl trinitrate
D   Ramipril
E   Simvastatin

2. A 68-year-old man is discharged from hospital following treatment for a non-ST-elevation myocardial infarction. He has made a good recovery and has no symptoms. His current medications are aspirin, clopidogrel, bisoprolol and atorvastatin.

What additional drug is most likely to reduce the risk of further cardiovascular events?

A   Amiloride
B   Digoxin
C   Glyceryl trinitrate
D   Ramipril
E   Warfarin

3. A 72-year-old man with a previous diagnosis of heart failure (New York Heart Association class III) complains of ankle swelling and is slightly more short of breath than usual. His current medications are bisoprolol, bumetanide and ramipril. Recent blood tests have showed mild hypokalaemia with a serum potassium concentration around 3.1 mmol/L (normal 3.5–4.7).

What drug should be added to his treatment?

A   Amiloride
B   Furosemide
C   Indapamide
D   Isosorbide mononitrate
E   Spironolactone

4. A 76-year-old man is found to have atrial fibrillation. He is asymptomatic. He has a past medical history of hypertension, hypercholesterolaemia and heart failure (New York Heart Association class II). He takes furosemide, ramipril and simvastatin, and has no allergies. Physical examination is normal except for a heart rate of approximately 120 beats/min with an irregular rhythm.

What is the most appropriate drug for ventricular rate control?

A   Amiodarone
B   Bisoprolol
C   Digoxin
D   Doxazosin
E   Verapamil

CVS

Mechanisms

5. An 82-year-old woman with ischaemic heart disease and cardiac failure is treated with bisoprolol, furosemide, ramipril, simvastatin and spironolactone.

Which of her medications acts by inhibiting a membrane transport protein?

A Bisoprolol
B Furosemide
C Ramipril ↙
D Simvastatin
E Spironolactone

CVS

Mechanisms

6. A 54-year-old man is found to have supraventricular tachycardia. He is treated with metoprolol in an attempt to terminate the arrhythmia.

What receptor is the main target of metoprolol?

A Alpha$_1$-adrenoceptor
B Alpha$_2$-adrenoceptor
C Beta$_1$-adrenoceptor
D Beta$_2$-adrenoceptor
E Beta$_3$-adrenoceptor

CVS

Interactions

7. An 81-year-old man presents with syncope. He has a past medical history of hypertension, angina and COPD. His usual oral medications are amlodipine, diltiazem, indapamide, ramipril and simvastatin. Two days ago he saw a doctor who did not have access to his full medical records, but advised him he should be taking a β-blocker. He prescribed bisoprolol.

On examination, his heart rate is 45 beats/min. His blood pressure is 96/60 mmHg. The ECG shows third-degree heart block.

What medication is interacting with bisoprolol to cause heart block?

A Amlodipine
B Diltiazem
C Indapamide
D Ramipril
E Simvastatin

CVS

Monitoring

8. A 58-year-old woman who started taking simvastatin 3 months ago is asked to attend a follow-up visit with her GP.

What blood test should be performed to monitor for side effects of statins?

A Creatine kinase
B Liver profile
C Fasting lipid profile
D Full blood count
E Thyroid function tests

CVS

Admin

9. A young man collapses at a wedding reception. He was seen fumbling with a cartridge-like device before he collapsed, but had not been able to use it. On examination, he is unresponsive. His breathing is noisy; this improves slightly with a head-tilt-chin-lift manoeuvre. His face appears flushed and his lips are swollen. A carotid pulse is palpable but it is thready.

An ambulance has been called but has not arrived. The cartridge-like device is handed to you. It is labelled 'EpiPen® Auto-Injector'.

How should this be administered?

A   Intramuscularly into the anterolateral thigh
B   Intramuscularly into the triceps muscle
C   Intravenously into any available peripheral vein
D   Subcutaneously into the anterior abdominal wall
E   Subcutaneously into the tissue overlying the triceps muscle

RS

Mechanisms

10. A 72-year-old man with hypertension, COPD and irritable bowel syndrome sees his GP for a medication review. His medicines are amlodipine, doxazocin, fluticasone, hyoscine butylbromide, ipratropium and salmeterol.

Which receptors have been activated by this treatment?

A   Alpha$_1$-adrenoceptors
B   Alpha$_2$-adrenoceptors
C   Beta$_1$-adrenoceptors
D   Beta$_2$-adrenoceptors
E   Muscarinic receptors

RS

Indications

11. A 12-year-old boy sees his general practitioner following hospital admission for an acute asthma attack. He has made a good recovery and is now asymptomatic.

What is the most appropriate treatment to prevent future asthma attacks?

A   Beclometasone
B   Formoterol
C   Chlorphenamine
D   Ipratropium
E   Salbutamol

RS

AEs

12. A 62-year-old man with COPD complains that one of his medications is causing a dry mouth. He is taking aminophylline, fluticasone, salbutamol, salmeterol and tiotropium.

What is the most likely cause of his dry mouth?

A   Aminophylline
B   Fluticasone
C   Salbutamol
D   Salmeterol
E   Tiotropium

NS
Indications

13. A 45-year-old woman is seen in her GP surgery with a 6-month history of moderate depression. Attempts to treat this with cognitive-behavioural therapy have proved unsuccessful. There are no psychotic features and she is assessed to be at low risk of self-harm. She has no other medical problems.

What is the most appropriate treatment?

A   Amitriptyline 25 mg daily
B   Citalopram 20 mg daily
C   Olanzapine 10 mg daily
D   Psychological interventions only
E   Mirtazapine 15 mg daily

NS
Indications
Prescription

14. A 40-year-old man is brought to the emergency department due to a fit. He is accompanied by a friend who says the fit started about 25 minutes ago. On examination, there are findings consistent with an ongoing clonic seizure. The capillary blood glucose concentration is 5.9 mmol/L. No antiepileptic treatment has been administered so far.

What is the most appropriate immediate treatment?

A   Carbamazepine 200 mg by nasogastric tube
B   Chlordiazepoxide 30 mg by nasogastric tube
C   Lorazepam 4 mg by slow IV injection
D   Phenytoin 20 mg/kg by IV infusion
E   Valproate 10 mg/kg by slow IV injection

NS
Warnings

15. A 34-year-old man presents to the emergency department following a tonic–clonic seizure. In the course of this he knocked over a kettle of boiling water and sustained a significant burn injury to his right arm, which will need to be cleaned once adequate analgesia is established. He had a past medical history of focal epilepsy, for which he takes carbamazepine.

What analgesic is most strongly contraindicated in this setting?

A   Codeine
B   Morphine
C   Naproxen
D   Paracetamol
E   Tramadol

GIS
Indications
Mechanisms
AEs

16. A 24-year-old woman is vomiting following an evacuation of retained products of conception (ERPC), performed under general anaesthesia. She was given cyclizine 50 mg IV 30 minutes ago but this has not improved her symptoms.

    Her past medical history is notable for a severe illness involving fever and muscles spasms, which was thought to have been precipitated by a prochlorperazine injection.

What is the most appropriate treatment for her nausea and vomiting?

A   Chlorpromazine
B   Cyclizine
C   Haloperidol
D   Metoclopramide
E   Ondansetron

GIS

Indications

Prescription

17. A 48-year-old woman who has peptic ulcers caused by *Helicobacter pylori* infection presents to her GP to commence treatment. She is allergic to benzylpenicillin, which caused an anaphylactic reaction.

What is the most appropriate 1-week oral treatment regimen?

A   Lansoprazole 30 mg 12-hourly, amoxicillin 1 g 12-hourly and clarithromycin 500 mg 12-hourly
B   Lansoprazole 30 mg 12-hourly, amoxicillin 1 g 12-hourly and metronidazole 400 mg 12-hourly
C   Omeprazole 20 mg 12-hourly and clarithromycin 500 mg 12-hourly
D   Omeprazole 20 mg 12-hourly and metronidazole 400 mg 8-hourly
E   Omeprazole 20 mg 12-hourly, clarithromycin 250 mg 12-hourly and metronidazole 400 mg 12-hourly

GIS

Indications

Mechanisms

18. An 86-year-old woman has been taking codeine phosphate to treat a sprained wrist. Co-incidentally, she has noticed that this improved the diarrhoea she usually suffers from as a result of diverticular disease.

Although her wrist has now healed, she is keen to continue taking the codeine, as not having to open her bowels so regularly has considerably improved her quality of life. However, the codeine does makes her feel a little 'light headed', which she finds unpleasant.

What alternative opioid would be better to treat her diarrhoea?

A   Loperamide
B   Morphine (immediate release)
C   Morphine (modified release)
D   Oxycodone (modified release)
E   Pethidine

GIS

Indications

19. A 62-year-old man with a background of alcoholic cirrhosis is admitted to the acute medical unit with confusion. A diagnosis of hepatic encephalopathy is made. His wife reports that he had been complaining of constipation in the days leading up to admission.

What laxative should be prescribed?

A   Docusate sodium
B   Ispaghula husk
C   Lactulose
D   Macrogol
E   Senna

20. A 50-year-old man complains of severe itch. He has had this for several days and it affects his whole body. He was admitted yesterday with progressive ascites due to cirrhotic liver disease. He is taking furosemide 40 mg orally daily, spironolactone 200 mg orally daily, lactulose 30 mL orally 8-hourly and phosphate enema 128 mL rectally daily. He has no allergies.

On examination of his skin, there are multiple spider naevi over his upper body and excoriation marks over his arms, trunk and thighs.

What is the most appropriate initial pharmacological treatment?

A   Chlorphenamine orally
B   Codeine phosphate orally
C   Hydrocortisone topically
D   Loratadine orally
E   Prednisolone orally

21. An 85-year-old woman is advised to take ranitidine for dyspepsia.

What best describes the mechanism of action of ranitidine?

A   Antagonism of histamine H_1 receptors in gastric parietal cells
B   Antagonism of histamine H_1 receptors in the vagus nerve
C   Antagonism of histamine H_2 receptors in gastric parietal cells
D   Antagonism of histamine H_2 receptors in gastric chief cells
E   Antagonism of histamine H_2 receptors in the vagus nerve

22. A 55-year-old woman with psoriatic arthritis was admitted to hospital 12 days ago with severe cellulitis. On admission her liver function was normal, but she has now developed cholestatic jaundice.

Her medications are flucloxacillin, methotrexate, morphine, paracetamol and simvastatin.

Which drug is most likely to have caused her cholestatic jaundice?

A   Flucloxacillin
B   Methotrexate
C   Morphine
D   Paracetamol
E   Simvastatin

23. A 72-year-old woman is found to be hypokalaemic. She had an elective right knee arthroplasty 3 days ago. Over the last 24 hours she has developed vomiting and abdominal pain. Viral gastroenteritis is suspected, as other patients on the ward have been affected by the same symptoms.

On examination, her pulse is 88 beats/min and her blood pressure is 156/90 mmHg. Her mucous membranes are dry. Her serum potassium concentration is 2.3 mmol/L (3.5–4.7). The rest of her serum biochemistry is normal. The ECG shows small T waves.

What is the most appropriate initial treatment?

A   Co-amilofruse 5/40 1 tablet orally

B   Potassium chloride 40 mmol in 1 L of sodium chloride 0.9% IV over 2 hours

C   Potassium chloride 40 mmol in 1 L of glucose 5% IV over 1 hour

D   Potassium chloride/bicarbonate (Sando-K®) 3 tablets orally

E   Ramipril 5 mg orally

24. A 73-year-old woman is advised to take oxybutynin to improve her symptoms of urinary urgency and urge incontinence.

What best describes the mechanism of action of oxybutynin?

A   Agonist at the β_2-adrenoceptor

B   Antagonist at the muscarinic M_3 receptor

C   Antagonist at the nicotinic acetylcholine receptor

D   Antagonist at the α_1-adrenoceptor

E   Inhibitor of 5α-reductase

25. A 48-year-old man is found to be hyperkalaemic. One month ago he was admitted to hospital with a non-ST-elevation myocardial infarction, for which he underwent percutaneous intervention. His medications, which were all started during the recent hospital admission, comprise aspirin, clopidogrel, atorvastatin, bisoprolol and ramipril.

What drug is most likely to cause hyperkalaemia?

A   Aspirin

B   Atorvastatin

C   Bisoprolol

D   Clopidogrel

E   Ramipril

Renal/GU

AEs

Indications

26. A 92-year-old woman, who lives in a residential home for people with dementia, is found confused and wandering. Her caregivers think that this was precipitated by a medicine for 'overactive bladder', which was started last week. Unfortunately they cannot find the drug in her room as she has been hiding things, and the GP surgery is closed.

What drug is most likely to have caused her confusion?

A   Finasteride
B   Furosemide
C   Solifenacin
D   Tamsulosin
E   Trimethoprim

Renal/GU

AEs

27. A 61-year-old man with benign prostatic hyperplasia is advised to take tamsulosin to improve urinary flow.

What side effect is most likely to occur when starting this new drug?

A   Bronchospasm
B   Postural hypotension
D   Erectile dysfunction
D   Gynaecomastia
E   Prostate cancer

Renal/GU

Warnings

28. An 82-year-old man with COPD is breathless and has recurrent exacerbations. His past medical history includes an episode of urinary retention secondary to benign prostatic hyperplasia.

Prescription of what drug requires a cautious approach in this patient?

A   Salbutamol
B   Salmeterol
C   Seretide®
D   Symbicort®
E   Tiotropium

Renal/GU

Infection

Warnings

29. A 33-year-old man with severe renal impairment requires antibiotic treatment for sepsis.

What antibiotic can generally be used without dosage reduction in severe renal impairment?

A   Benzylpenicillin
B   Co-amoxiclav
C   Doxycycline
D   Gentamicin
E   Metronidazole

30. A 67-year-old man presents to the general practice to discuss his medication. For several years he has been taking sildenafil for erectile dysfunction. He has previously found this to be an effective and tolerable treatment, but says it has recently been causing headaches.

He has a past medical history of chronic obstructive pulmonary disease. In addition, he was recently found to have atrial fibrillation. His treatment has been adjusted frequently over the past few weeks. His regular treatment now comprises digoxin, diltiazem, simvastatin, tiotropium and warfarin. Examination is normal other than for an irregular pulse at a rate of 80–90 beats/min.

What drug is most likely to interact with sildenafil to provoke side effects?

A   Digoxin
B   Diltiazem
C   Simvastatin
D   Tiotropium
E   Warfarin

31. A 66-year-old woman with severe chronic pain takes amitriptyline, ibuprofen, morphine, omeprazole and senna.

Which of her medications acts by enzyme inhibition?

A   Amitriptyline
B   Ibuprofen
C   Morphine
D   Omeprazole
E   Senna

32. A 63-year-old man with gout, hypertension and hypercholesterolaemia complains of swelling and pain in his left big toe. His GP makes a diagnosis of acute gout. His regular medications are allopurinol, amlodipine, indapamide, ramipril and simvastatin.

What drug could be stopped or substituted to reduce the risk of future attacks of gout?

A   Allopurinol
B   Amlodipine
C   Indapamide
D   Ramipril
E   Simvastatin

MSK
Poisoning
AEs

33. A 63-year-old woman, who is an inpatient, complains of headache, nausea and sore mouth. She was admitted 2 weeks ago with a fracture of her left femoral neck. She has a past medical history of rheumatoid arthritis.

Blood tests reveal new renal and liver impairment and pancytopenia. Reviewing her drug chart, you notice that her methotrexate has been prescribed daily instead of weekly.

What is the most appropriate immediate treatment for her methotrexate toxicity?

A   Activated charcoal
B   Folic acid
C   Folinic acid
D   Granulocyte stimulating factor (G-CSF)
E   Haemodialysis

Blood
Indications
Prescription

34. An 85-year-old woman is admitted to the acute medical unit with a urinary tract infection. Her past medical history includes a left-leg deep vein thrombosis 5 years ago, for which she was treated with warfarin for 3 months. She has no risk factors for bleeding and her renal function is normal.

What is the most appropriate antithrombotic therapy while in hospital?

A   Aspirin 75 mg orally daily
B   Dalteparin 5000 units SC daily
C   Dalteparin 5000 units SC daily and warfarin orally to target INR 2–3
D   Unfractionated heparin 5000 units SC 12-hourly
E   Warfarin orally to target INR 2–3

Blood
Interactions

35. A 77-year-old woman attends the anticoagulation clinic. She has a past medical history of atrial fibrillation and stroke. She takes warfarin and has been on a stable dosage for about 2 years. Last month, she was briefly admitted to hospital following a seizure. This was ascribed to cerebrovascular disease and she was put on an 'antiepileptic medicine'. She does not know its name and has not brought a list of her medications.

Her INR today is 1.6 (target 2–3).

What drug is most likely to interact with warfarin to lower the INR?

A   Carbamazepine
B   Diazepam
C   Gabapentin
D   Pregabalin
E   Valproate

Infection
Renal/GU
Indications
Warnings

36. A 22-year-old woman complains of dysuria. Her GP diagnoses an uncomplicated urinary tract infection. Her only medication is the combined oral contraceptive pill and she has not missed any doses of this. She has no allergies.

What is the most appropriate treatment?

A   Cefotaxime
B   Ciprofloxacin
C   Clarithromycin
D   Gentamicin
E   Trimethoprim

Infection
Skin
Indications

37. A 72-year-old woman is admitted to hospital with severe cellulitis of her right leg. She has no allergies.

What is the most appropriate treatment?

A   Amoxicillin and clarithromycin
B   Benzylpenicillin and flucloxacillin
C   Cefotaxime and aciclovir
D   Co-amoxiclav and metronidazole
E   Co-amoxiclav and gentamicin

Infection
RS
Indications

38. An 83-year-old woman is admitted to the acute medical unit with a diagnosis of mild community-acquired pneumonia (CURB-65 score 1). Her mobility is poor, but she has no active co-morbidities, does not usually take any medications, and has no allergies.

What would be the most appropriate antibiotic to treat her infection?

A   Cefotaxime
B   Ciprofloxacin
C   Doxycycline
D   Ertapenem
E   Flucloxacillin

Infection
Mechanisms

39. A 44-year-old man needs antibiotic treatment for infection with a penicillinase-producing strain of *Staphylococcus aureus*.

What antibiotic is this organism most likely to be resistant to?

A   Benzylpenicillin
B   Co-amoxiclav
C   Flucloxacillin
D   Tazocin®
E   Vancomycin

Infection

NS

AEs

40. A 56-year-old man notices tinnitus and dizziness after discharge from hospital where he was treated for severe pneumonia. During this admission (which included a spell in the intensive care unit), his antibiotic treatment included courses of doxycycline, co-amoxiclav, clarithromycin, piperacillin with tazobactam, and gentamicin.

Which antibiotic is most likely to have caused this adverse effect?

A   Clarithromycin
B   Co-amoxiclav
C   Doxycycline
D   Gentamicin
E   Piperacillin with tazobactam

Infection

RS

Warnings

41. A 4-year-old boy is found to have pneumonia.

What antibiotic is contraindicated at this age?

A   Amoxicillin
B   Cefotaxime
C   Co-amoxiclav
D   Clarithromycin
E   Doxycycline

Infection

CVS

AEs

42. A 68-year-old woman is found to have cellulitis. She has a past medical history of hypertension, leg cramps and urge incontinence. Her medication comprises bendroflumethiazide, oxybutynin and quinine sulfate. She is allergic to penicillin, which causes a rash. The doctor begins to prescribe clarithromycin, but is alerted to a possible interaction by the electronic prescribing system.

What is the main risk of prescribing clarithromycin in this case?

A   Hyperkalaemia
B   QT-interval prolongation
C   Renal impairment
D   Myopathy
E   Seizures

Infection

RS

Interactions

Comm

43. A 72-year-old woman is advised to take doxycycline 100 mg daily and prednisolone 30 mg daily for an exacerbation of chronic obstructive pulmonary disease. Her usual medication is aspirin 75 mg daily, ferrous sulfate 200 mg twice daily, furosemide 40 mg daily, lansoprazole 30 mg daily, and ramipril 5 mg daily.

What medicine should she be advised to separate from doxycycline by at least 2 hours?

A   Aspirin
B   Ferrous sulfate
C   Furosemide
D   Lansoprazole
E   Ramipril

Infection

Admin

44. A 92-year-old man with severe fluid overload requires treatment with intravenous antibiotics. The cardiologist has recommended that these be given as low volume bolus injections rather than by infusion if possible.

Which antibiotic can be administered as an intravenous bolus injection?

A   Amoxicillin
B   Clarithromycin
C   Doxycycline
D   Gentamicin
E   Vancomycin

Infection

Interactions

Comm

45. A 29-year-old man who has been advised to take antibiotics asks his doctor if he can drink alcohol while on treatment.

What antibiotic should not be taken with alcohol?

A   Amoxicillin
B   Clarithromycin
C   Doxycycline
D   Metronidazole
E   Trimethoprim

Infection

Renal/GU

Monitoring

46. A 47-year-old woman is being treated with once daily gentamicin for pyelonephritis. She received her first dose 21 hours ago. Her next dose is due in 3 hours and the nurse has called you to ask if any tests need to be performed before it is given.

What test should be performed 18–24 hours after the first dose of gentamicin?

A   Audiometry
B   C-reactive protein concentration
C   Estimated glomerular filtration rate
D   Serum creatinine concentration
E   Serum gentamicin concentration

Poisoning

Indications

47. A 31-year-old man presents 7 hours after a paracetamol overdose. His only symptoms are nausea and epigastric discomfort. He has no relevant past medical history and takes no regular medication. The serum paracetamol concentration is above the treatment line on the paracetamol poisoning treatment graph.

What is the most appropriate treatment?

A   Acetylcysteine
B   Activated charcoal
C   Cyclizine
D   Omeprazole
E   Naloxone

48. A 24-year-old woman is receiving an intravenous infusion of acetylcysteine for paracetamol poisoning. Thirty minutes into the infusion, she develops a rash. On examination, her heart rate is 95 beats/min and her blood pressure is 117/78 mmHg. She has a widespread urticarial rash.

What is the most appropriate immediate management?

A   Continue acetylcysteine and give chlorphenamine
B   Continue acetylcysteine and give ranitidine
C   Temporarily stop acetylcysteine and give adrenaline
D   Temporarily stop acetylcysteine and give chlorphenamine
E   Temporarily stop acetylcysteine and give ranitidine

49. A 75-year-old man is admitted 1 hour after an acute ischaemic stroke. He is aphasic and his swallow is judged to be unsafe. It has not been possible to insert a nasogastric tube. You are asked to prescribe intravenous fluid to cover the next 24–36 hours.

He weighs 80 kg. He is not dehydrated. His serum potassium concentration and renal function are normal.

What is the most appropriate fluid regimen to prescribe at this stage?

A   500 mL glucose 5% over 12 h
    500 mL sodium chloride 0.9% over 12 h

B   1 L glucose 5% over 12 h
    1 L sodium chloride 0.9% over 12 h

C   1 L sodium chloride 0.9% over 10 h
    1 L sodium chloride 0.9% over 10 h
    1 L glucose 5% with potassium chloride 40 mmol over 10 h

D   1 L glucose 5% with potassium chloride 40 mmol over 8 h
    1 L glucose 5% with potassium chloride 40 mmol over 8 h
    500 mL sodium chloride 0.9% over 8 h

E   1 L glucose 5% with potassium chloride 20 mmol over 8 h
    1 L glucose 5% with potassium chloride 20 mmol over 8 h
    1 L glucose 5% with potassium chloride 20 mmol over 8 h

Fluids

Indications

Prescription

50. A 35-year-old woman is found to be hypotensive. She was admitted 6 hours ago with acute pancreatitis. Analgesia and intravenous fluids were administered and she was transferred to the ward. Over the past hour, her heart rate has been 100–110 beats/min and her blood pressure around 85/50 mmHg She has not passed any urine since admission. Her serum potassium concentration is 5.1 mmol/L (normal 3.5–4.7).

What is the most appropriate option for initial fluid resuscitation?

A   Compound sodium lactate (Hartmann's solution) 500 mL IV over 10 minutes

B   Glucose 5% 500 mL IV over 10 minutes

C   Human albumin solution 5% 250 mL IV over 10 minutes

D   Sodium chloride 0.9% 500 mL IV over 10 minutes

E   Sterile water 500 mL IV over 10 minutes

Answers and explanations

1. B. Bisoprolol. Angina occurs when insufficient blood is able to pass through narrowed atheromatous coronary arteries to meet myocardial oxygen demand. Beta-blockers, such as bisoprolol, are first choice drugs for the prevention of angina. They work by slowing the heart rate and reducing cardiac contractility, which in turn reduces myocardial work and oxygen demand. Calcium channel blockers and long-acting nitrates are alternatives. Short-acting nitrates, such as glyceryl trinitrate, are taken during an attack of angina to relieve chest pain. They can be taken before exercise to reduce the risk of angina, but are less effective in preventing angina than regularly-administered alternatives.

Aspirin, ACE inhibitors and statins do not directly prevent angina. A statin should be offered to all patients with ischaemic heart disease to reduce the risk of future coronary events. ACE inhibitors and aspirin should be offered to people who have atherosclerotic disease (e.g. ischaemic heart disease, cerebrovascular disease) to reduce the risk of recurrent events or death.

2. D. Ramipril. Clinical trials have shown that ACE inhibitors such as ramipril, antiplatelet agents (e.g. aspirin, clopidogrel), β-blockers and statins significantly reduce the risk of recurrent events or death following a myocardial infarction. These drugs should be prescribed in combination for secondary prevention of cardiovascular events in all patients following myocardial infarction unless contraindicated.

The other drugs have no role in secondary prevention following myocardial infarction. Amiloride is a potassium-sparing diuretic, used to reduce potassium losses in patients taking other diuretics (loop or thiazide diuretics). Digoxin is a cardiac glycoside. It is an option for rate control in atrial fibrillation, particularly in people with heart failure. Glyceryl trinitrate is a nitrate which is used to relieve angina by reducing myocardial work and oxygen demand; however, it does not prevent myocardial infarction. Warfarin is an anticoagulant. It is used to reduce the risk of intracardiac thrombus formation and of systemic embolism in patients with atrial fibrillation.

3. E. Spironolactone. This patient needs treatment to control his symptoms of heart failure (ankle swelling and shortness of breath), and to normalise his serum potassium concentration, since hypokalaemia is associated with a risk of dangerous arrhythmias. Aldosterone antagonists, such as spironolactone, competitively block the aldosterone receptor, causing increased sodium and water excretion and potassium retention in the distal renal tubules. Although aldosterone antagonists are relatively weak diuretics, they can improve symptoms and reduce mortality in patients with moderate heart failure. They also increase the serum potassium concentration.

Furosemide (a loop diuretic, like bumetanide which he is already taking) and indapamide (a thiazide-like diuretic) could improve symptoms by increasing sodium and water excretion. However, both drugs may further reduce the serum potassium concentration by increasing renal potassium excretion. Nitrates are used in the treatment of acute, but not chronic, heart failure and will not address the hypokalaemia. Amiloride (a potassium-sparing diuretic) can increase the serum potassium concentration but is a weak diuretic that will have little impact on symptoms and offers no prognostic benefits in heart failure.

4. B. Bisoprolol. There are two basic approaches to managing chronic atrial fibrillation. One is 'rhythm control', which seeks to restore normal sinus rhythm either by electrical cardioversion, antiarrhythmic drugs, or both. The other is 'rate control', in which the abnormal heart rhythm is accepted as permanent, and efforts are focused simply on preventing ventricular rate from running too fast. In most cases, rate control is just as effective as rhythm control and considerably simpler.

The ideal agent for ventricular rate control in atrial fibrillation is either a β-blocker (e.g. bisoprolol) or a non-dihydropyridine calcium channel blocker (e.g. verapamil or diltiazem). In practice, a β-blocker is used in most patients. This would be a particularly appropriate choice for this patient due to his history of heart failure: β-blockers are indicated in heart failure to improve prognosis, whereas verapamil and diltiazem should be avoided.

Digoxin can be used for rate control in atrial fibrillation but, on its own, it is less effective than a β-blocker or calcium channel blocker and potentially more toxic. Likewise, although amiodarone is an effective agent for both rate and rhythm control in atrial fibrillation, it is much too toxic for first-line use. Doxazosin is an α-blocker used in hypertension and benign prostatic hyperplasia; it has no role in atrial fibrillation.

5. B. Furosemide. Furosemide is a loop diuretic which inhibits the $Na^+/K^+/2Cl^-$ co-transporter in the ascending loop of Henle, preventing transport of sodium, potassium and chloride ions from the renal tubular lumen into the epithelial cell.

Bisoprolol and spironolactone are receptor antagonists that block β₁-adrenoceptors and aldosterone receptors, respectively (see Beta-blockers and Aldosterone antagonists). Ramipril and simvastatin are enzyme inhibitors. Ramipril is an angiotensin converting enzyme (ACE) inhibitor, preventing conversion of angiotensin I to angiotensin II. Simvastatin, a statin, inhibits HMG Co-A reductase, preventing the synthesis of cholesterol.

6. C. Beta₁ adrenoceptor. Metoprolol is a β-blocker that is relatively selective for the β₁-adrenoceptor. Blockade of this receptor reduces force of myocardial contraction and decreases the speed of electrical conduction in the heart. By prolonging the refractory period of the atrioventricular node and slowing conduction in the atria, it can terminate some supraventricular tachycardias and reduce the ventricular rate in atrial fibrillation.

Beta₂-adrenoceptors are found in smooth muscle, such as in the bronchial tree; β₃-adrenoceptors are found in adipose tissue. Blockade of these receptors is not clinically useful in the management of supraventricular tachycardias such as atrial fibrillation. Metoprolol does not have any effect on α-adrenoceptors.

7. B. Diltiazem. Diltiazem, like verapamil, is a non-dihydropyridine <u>calcium channel blocker</u>. Non-dihydropyridine calcium channel blockers are relatively cardioselective: they reduce the rate and force of cardiac contraction, and interfere with conduction at the atrioventricular node. These effects are similar to those of β-blockers. Non-dihydropyridine calcium channel blockers and β-blockers should not be combined except under the close supervision of a specialist, as their effects on the heart are additive. Together, they can cause heart block, cardiogenic shock, and even asystole. This patient has third-degree heart block. That is, transmission between the atria and ventricles is completely blocked and they are now beating independently. This serious interaction highlights the dangers of prescribing drugs without a full and accurate medication history.

Amlodipine is a dihydropyridine calcium channel blocker. In contrast to diltiazem, its effects are principally on the blood vessels, where it causes vasodilation. Its effects on cardiac conduction and contractility are minimal. Indapamide is a <u>thiazide-like diuretic</u> and ramipril is an <u>ACE inhibitor</u>. These drugs have no direct effect on cardiac conduction or contractility. Amlodipine, indapamide and ramipril can all be combined with a β-blocker provided the hypotensive effect is not prohibitive. Simvastatin, a <u>statin</u>, does not interact with β-blockers.

8. B. Liver profile. Around 1 in 200 patients taking a <u>statin</u> will develop elevated liver enzymes or significant muscle side effects (myopathy, rhabdomyolysis). Early detection of this allows treatment to be adjusted, minimising the risk of long-term harm. A liver profile should be measured before starting statin treatment and again at 3 months. The statin should be stopped if liver transaminase levels increase to greater than three times the upper limit of normal.

Patients should be advised to report new muscle aches and pains to their doctor. However, there is no need to check creatine kinase levels unless these occur. Thyroid function should be checked *before* a statin is started, as untreated hypothyroidism is a reversible cause of hyperlipidaemia and can increase the risk of adverse effects from statins. A lipid profile may be a useful marker of *efficacy*, rather than safety, although in current guidelines target levels are specified only for secondary prevention.

9. A. Intramuscularly into the anterolateral thigh. <u>Adrenaline</u> is the most important treatment for anaphylaxis. People who have experienced an anaphylactic reaction should be provided with an adrenaline auto-injector for self-administration in the event of a recurrent attack. The EpiPen® (adult form) is designed to deliver 300 micrograms of adrenaline as an intramuscular injection. It should be administered into the anterolateral thigh. You do this by removing the blue safety cap then jabbing the orange end of the device firmly against the outer thigh, holding it there for about 10 seconds. It can be given through clothing if necessary. Of note, not all the contents of the glass cartridge will be injected; the device contains 2 mg of adrenaline (as a 1 mg/mL solution) and delivers only 0.3 mg (0.3 mL) of this.

Injection into smaller muscles is less desirable as absorption is not as reliable, but they can be used if necessary. The subcutaneous route should not be used as absorption is too slow. Adrenaline must not be administered intravenously unless cardiac arrest supervenes.

10. D. Beta₂-adrenoceptors. Beta₂-adrenoceptors are activated by salmeterol, a long-acting β_2-agonist bronchodilator.

Doxazocin is an α-blocker, which antagonises α_1-adrenoceptors. Ipratropium and hyoscine butylbromide block muscarinic receptors (see Antimuscarinics, bronchodilators and Antimuscarinics, cardiovascular and gastrointestinal uses, respectively). Amlodipine is a calcium channel blocker. Fluticasone is an inhaled corticosteroid which activates glucocorticoid receptors to influence gene transcription.

11. A. Beclometasone. Corticosteroids such as beclometasone suppress inflammation in the airways, reducing the risk of asthma attacks. Topical administration by inhaler reduces systemic side effects.

Ipratropium (an antimuscarinic) and salbutamol (a β_2-agonist) are short-acting bronchodilators. They are used to relieve breathlessness in acute attacks. They may also be taken before activities that are expected to provoke symptoms, such as exercise. However, they have no role as a regular treatment to prevent attacks. Formoterol is a long-acting β_2-agonist. It is taken regularly to improve lung function, but it does not address the underlying pathology (inflammation). For this reason, it must not be given without an inhaled corticosteroid, so would be an inappropriate choice at this stage. Antihistamines (e.g. chlorphenamine) can improve symptoms of histamine-mediated allergic disease such as hayfever and skin itching, but do not prevent or control airways inflammation in asthma.

12. E. Tiotropium. Tiotropium is a long-acting antimuscarinic bronchodilator which inhibits parasympathetic stimulation of salivation, causing a dry mouth. None of the other drugs listed cause a dry mouth, although inhaled fluticasone (an inhaled corticosteroid) can cause oral thrush, the risk of which is reduced by rinsing and gargling after inhalation.

13. B. Citalopram 20 mg daily. Antidepressants are indicated for moderate and severe depression, and for mild depression that has not responded adequately to psychological interventions, as in this case. A selective-serotonin re-uptake inhibitor (SSRI), such as citalopram, is first choice in most patients. Amitriptyline (a tricyclic antidepressant) and mirtazapine (an antagonist of pre-synaptic α_2-adrenoceptors) are also effective antidepressants, but as they cause more side effects they are generally reserved for cases in which SSRIs are deemed unsuitable. Olanzapine is a second-generation antipsychotic which is not indicated for non-psychotic depression.

14. C. Lorazepam 4 mg by slow IV injection. Broadly, status epilepticus may be defined as a state of unrelenting seizure activity. It is a life-threatening condition that requires urgent treatment. First-line pharmacological treatment is with a benzodiazepine, which in a hospital setting should be administered intravenously. The ideal choice is lorazepam due to its long duration of effect. In adults, this is usually given in an initial dose of 4 mg by slow IV injection, which may be repeated once if the seizure does not terminate. Diazepam is a reasonable alternative if lorazepam is unavailable. Chlordiazepoxide is also a long-acting benzodiazepine, ut it is not available in an intravenous formulation so is not suited to use in status epilepticus. If the seizure cannot be controlled with a benzodiazepine, the antiepileptic drug <u>phenytoin</u> may be given. If this is unsuccessful, the patient should be anaesthetised and managed in the intensive care unit.

<u>Valproate</u> and <u>carbamazepine</u> are alternative antiepileptic drugs. In the context of status epilepticus, valproate is sometimes used in place of phenytoin as a second-line agent. <u>Carbamazepine</u> has no role in the acute management of status epilepticus.

15. E. Tramadol. You need to be particularly careful when prescribing for patients with epilepsy, for two main reasons. Firstly, antiepileptic drugs (including <u>phenytoin</u>, <u>carbamazepine</u> and <u>valproate</u>) have many potential drug interactions. These may result in drug toxicity (either of the antiepileptic drug or the other interacting drug) or loss of seizure control. Secondly, there are a number of drugs that can lower the seizure threshold, including <u>antidepressants</u>, <u>antipsychotics</u>, and <u>opioids</u>, particularly tramadol. The other opioids may have an effect on seizure threshold, but this is much less significant. In the context of severe pain, their benefits are likely to outweigh their risks. Naproxen (an <u>NSAID</u>) and <u>paracetamol</u> are not known to affect seizure threshold or interact with carbamazepine.

16. E. Ondansetron. Predicting which antiemetic will work in which patient is not easy. In practice, drug selection is often based on pragmatic considerations such as familiarity and availability, and then adjusted according to the patient's response. With her having already had cyclizine (an <u>antiemetic</u> that acts by <u>histamine H_1-receptor antagonism</u>), it would now be best to offer a drug from a different class. This choice is influenced by her past reaction to prochlorperazine, which sounds like neuroleptic malignant syndrome (NMS). NMS is a serious condition that may be precipitated by drugs that have an anti-dopaminergic effect, including <u>phenothiazine antiemetics</u> (e.g. prochlorperazine, chlorpromazine), <u>dopamine antagonist antiemetics</u> (e.g. metoclopramide) and <u>antipsychotics</u> (including haloperidol, which is sometimes also used as an antiemetic). The risk of recurrence of NMS with re-exposure is unclear, but it would be prudent to avoid these drug classes where suitable alternatives exist. Ondansetron is an antiemetic that works by <u>serotonin 5-HT_3-receptor antagonism</u>; it is not associated with NMS.

17. E. Omeprazole 20 mg 12-hourly, clarithromycin 250 mg 12-hourly and metronidazole 400 mg 12-hourly. *Helicobacter pylori* is a Gram-negative bacterium which causes peptic ulcer disease. Effective treatment requires combination therapy with two antibiotics and a <u>proton pump inhibitor</u> for 1 week. Treatment with a single antibiotic may be ineffective and may cause the bacteria to develop resistance.

The various regimens considered acceptable for *H. pylori* eradication, including recommended drug doses, are set out in a helpful table in the British National Formulary. Options for proton pump inhibition include lansoprazole, omeprazole and pantoprazole. The antibiotics are selected from amoxicillin (a <u>broad-spectrum penicillin</u>), clarithromycin (a <u>macrolide</u>) and <u>metronidazole</u>. As this patient has previously had an anaphylactic reaction to benzylpenicillin, amoxicillin is contraindicated and clarithromycin with metronidazole should be used. You should note that the doses recommended for antibiotics when used in *H. pylori* eradication may differ from those used in other indications.

18. A. Loperamide. Loperamide is an <u>antimotility drug</u> used in selected cases of diarrhoea. Pharmacologically, it is an <u>opioid</u> similar to pethidine, but unlike other opioids it does not cross the blood–brain barrier. This means it is devoid of central nervous system effects, including analgesia, but retains the peripheral effects such as reducing gut motility. The antimotility effects are mediated by opioid μ-receptor agonism in the myenteric plexus of the gastrointestinal tract.

While the other opioids in this list will have similar antimotility effects, they are likely also to cause central nervous system effects which, in this context, are undesirable.

19. C. Lactulose. One of the main substances involved in the pathogenesis of hepatic encephalopathy is ammonia. Lactulose is an <u>osmotic laxative</u> that reduces absorption of ammonia by increasing transit rate of colonic contents and by acidifying the stool, which inhibits the proliferation of ammonia-producing bacteria. This makes it an important treatment for patients with, or at risk of, hepatic encephalopathy, regardless of whether they are constipated. In these circumstances, the aim should be for patients to produce three loose stools each day. The other drugs are all laxatives that will treat his constipation but will not be as beneficial in treating his encephalopathy.

20. D. Loratadine orally. Pruritus is a common problem in liver disease. Non pharmacological measures such as warm baths may be helpful but are often insufficient. First-line pharmacological treatment is usually with an <u>antihistamine</u>. When prescribing for patients with advanced liver disease, it is important to avoid using sedating drugs wherever possible. This is because sedation can precipitate hepatic encephalopathy. Chlorphenamine is a first-generation antihistamine with pronounced sedative effects. By contrast, loratadine is a second-generation antihistamine which, by virtue of not crossing the blood–brain barrier, does not cause sedation.

<u>Topical corticosteroids</u> are sometimes used for inflammatory lesions associated with pruritus (e.g. eczema), but they are not an option for generalised pruritus. <u>Systemic corticosteroids</u> are not used for pruritus. As an <u>opioid</u> agonist, codeine phosphate may *cause* itch. Furthermore, its sedative effects may be problematic.

21. C. Antagonism of histamine H_2 receptors in gastric parietal cells.
Ranitidine is a <u>histamine H_2-receptor blocker</u>. Histamine is released from paracrine cells in the stomach and binds to H_2-receptors on gastric parietal cell walls. Acting through second messenger systems, this activates the proton pumps that are responsible for gastric acid secretion. By blocking H_2 receptors, ranitidine increases the pH of the stomach contents and thereby reduces symptoms of gastritis and gastro-oesophageal reflux.

22. A. Flucloxacillin. Cholestatic jaundice is a rare, but potentially serious, adverse effect of flucloxacillin (a penicillinase-resistant penicillin). It can occur even when treatment has been completed and is a contraindication to future use of this drug.

Although paracetamol, methotrexate and simvastatin (a statin) can all cause liver toxicity, they do not generally cause cholestatic jaundice. Paracetamol in overdose causes hepatocellular necrosis, which can be fatal if untreated. Methotrexate can cause hepatitis as part of a hypersensitivity reaction or if taken in overdose. Chronic use of methotrexate can cause hepatic cirrhosis. Statins can cause a rise in liver enzymes (transaminases) and, less frequently, drug-induced hepatitis. Morphine does not cause hepatotoxicity, but it is metabolised in the liver so dose reduction is required in people with liver failure.

23. B. Potassium chloride 40 mmol in 1 L of sodium chloride 0.9% IV over 2 hours. Hypokalaemia is a potentially dangerous electrolyte abnormality due to its association with arrhythmias. A serum potassium concentration <2.5 mmol/L is generally deemed to be 'severe', and this warrants intravenous treatment. In a general ward environment, this is administered through a peripheral cannula using a potassium-containing fluid. Option B, containing potassium chloride 40 mmol/L, is a reasonable choice.

Option A is a combination of a loop diuretic (furosemide) and a potassium-sparing diuretic (amiloride). If hypokalaemia occurs during treatment with furosemide, exchanging it for co-amilofruse may resolve this. It is not suitable for treatment of other causes of hypokalaemia. Option C is inappropriate because the rate of intravenous potassium administration is too fast: it should not exceed 20 mmol/hr on a general ward. Also, it is usually better to treat hypokalaemia using a sodium-chloride-based fluid than glucose (see Potassium, intravenous). Option D, potassium orally, is the preferred treatment for *non-severe* hypokalaemia. Option E, an ACE inhibitor, does have a potassium-elevating effect. However, it is not an appropriate treatment for acute hypokalaemia. Indeed, ACE inhibitors should be avoided whenever there is a risk of acute kidney injury, such as in patients who have become dehydrated.

24. B. Antagonist at the muscarinic M_3 receptor. Oxybutynin is an antimuscarinic drug that preferentially blocks the M_3 receptor in the bladder. This inhibits the procontractile effect of parasympathetic stimulation, causing relaxation of the bladder smooth muscle and increasing bladder capacity. This makes it a useful option for treatment for urge incontinence and overactive bladder symptoms.

Alpha$_1$-blockers (e.g. doxazosin) and 5α-reductase inhibitors (e.g. finasteride) are used to treat symptoms of benign prostatic hyperplasia. They have no role in the treatment of overactive bladder. Beta$_2$-agonists are used to induce smooth muscle relaxation in the airways; they are not used for overactive bladder. The nicotinic acetylcholine receptor is involved in neuromuscular transmission in skeletal muscle. Antagonists of this receptor are used in anaesthetic practice to induce muscle relaxation.

25. E. Ramipril. <u>ACE inhibitors</u> (e.g. ramipril) commonly cause an increase in the serum potassium concentration. This can usually be tolerated provided it does not exceed 6.0 mmol/L. Other drugs with a significant potassium-elevating effect include <u>angiotensin-receptor blockers</u>, <u>aldosterone-receptor antagonists</u>, oral and intravenous <u>potassium</u> supplements, and <u>potassium-sparing diuretics</u>. <u>Beta-blockers</u> and <u>aspirin</u> can also increase the potassium concentration, but this effect is not usually significant. <u>Statins</u> and <u>clopidogrel</u> do not cause hyperkalaemia.

26. C. Solifenacin. Solifenacin is an <u>antimuscarinic</u> drug used to treat urinary urgency and urge incontinence. Side effects of antimuscarinics include dry mouth, blurred vision, constipation and confusion. Elderly patients, especially those with dementia, are particularly vulnerable to these side effects. The reasons for susceptibility to confusion are complex but include alteration in drug distribution and metabolism as well as increased sensitivity to their central nervous system effects. Where possible, alternative therapies should be used.

The other drugs listed are unlikely to have been started in this case. Finasteride is a <u>5α-reductase inhibitor</u> and tamsulosin is an <u>α-blocker</u>; they are both used in men with benign prostatic hyperplasia, but not in overactive bladder. They are not known to cause confusion. Furosemide is a <u>loop diuretic</u> used in states of fluid overload such as heart failure, and does not directly cause confusion (although over-diuresis leading to dehydration might). <u>Trimethoprim</u> is an antibiotic that acts by interfering with bacterial folate synthesis. It is commonly used to treat urinary tract infections, but not overactive bladder. It causes confusion very rarely.

27. B. Postural hypotension. Tamsulosin (an <u>α-blocker</u>) blocks α_1-adrenoceptors in the smooth muscle of the prostate gland, increasing urinary flow and relieving obstructive symptoms. As α_1-adrenoceptors are also found in the smooth muscle of blood vessels, α-blockers can cause hypotension, particularly postural hypotension. Patients taking other antihypertensive medication should be especially vigilant to these effects and may need to omit their usual treatment when starting an α-blocker. Bronchospasm and erectile dysfunction are adverse effects of <u>β-blockers</u> (not α-blockers). Tamsulosin does not cause gynaecomastia or prostate cancer.

28. E. Tiotropium. Tiotropium is a long-acting <u>antimuscarinic bronchodilator</u>. Its side effects include urinary retention in people susceptible to this. It should therefore be avoided or used cautiously in patients with a history of urinary retention, or risk factors such as benign prostatic hyperplasia.

Salbutamol and salmeterol are, respectively, short- and long-acting <u>β_2-agonists</u>. Seretide® and Symbicort® are <u>compound β_2-agonist–corticosteroid inhalers</u>. Warnings regarding their use can be reviewed under the relevant individual drug entries.

29. E. Metronidazole. <u>Metronidazole</u> is metabolised and eliminated by the liver. Dosage reduction is therefore required in severe hepatic impairment rather than renal impairment.

Many other antibiotics are eliminated by the kidney. In patients with renal impairment they may therefore accumulate, increasing the risk of adverse effects. However, there is always a balance to be struck between the risk of drug toxicity and the risk of undertreating the infection. As such, renal impairment does not necessarily contraindicate the drugs' use, but it does mandate a more cautious approach to drug selection and dosing regimens.

In severe renal impairment, dose reductions are required with <u>penicillins</u> such as benzylpenicillin and co-amoxiclav due to the risk of central nervous system toxicity, including fits; <u>tetracyclines</u> such as doxycycline due to the risk of hepatotoxicity and nephrotoxicity; and <u>aminoglycosides</u> such as gentamicin, which may cause ototoxicity and nephrotoxicity.

30. B. Diltiazem. Sildenafil is a <u>phosphodiesterase (type 5) inhibitor</u>. It is metabolised by a member of the cytochrome P450 enzyme family called CYP3A4. Diltiazem is a <u>calcium channel blocker</u> that inhibits CYP3A4 activity. If the drugs are taken together, the metabolism of sildenafil will be reduced such that the patient is exposed to higher sildenafil concentrations. This increases the chance of dose-related adverse effects, such as headache. A reduced dose of sildenafil is recommended in patients taking cytochrome P450 inhibitors, other examples of which include <u>amiodarone</u> and <u>macrolide antibiotics</u>.

Diltiazem can also interact with digoxin, since they both reduce conduction at the atrioventricular node. This interaction may be exploited therapeutically, as in this case, to slow the ventricular rate in patients with atrial fibrillation. There are no other clinically significant interactions between the drugs listed.

31. B. Ibuprofen. Ibuprofen is a <u>non-steroidal anti-inflammatory drug</u> (NSAID), which inhibits the enzyme cyclooxygenase, preventing conversion of arachidonic acid to prostaglandins.

Amitriptyline and omeprazole inhibit membrane transport proteins. Amitriptyline is a <u>tricyclic antidepressant</u> that inhibits transporters responsible for removing serotonin and noradrenaline from the synaptic cleft. Omeprazole is a <u>proton pump inhibitor</u> that inhibits H^+/K^+-ATPase in gastric parietal cells, preventing the secretion of gastric acid. Morphine is a <u>strong opioid</u> that activates opioid μ (mu) receptors in the central nervous system. Senna is a <u>stimulant laxative</u> that acts as an irritant in the gut to increase water and electrolyte secretion from the colonic mucosa.

32. C. Indapamide. Gout is caused by deposition of uric acid in joints. The first metatarsophalangeal joint (of the big toe) is the most commonly affected site. The likely precipitant in this patient is indapamide, a <u>thiazide-like diuretic</u>, which reduces uric acid excretion by the kidneys. Other drug causes of gout include *low-dose aspirin*, some anti-cancer drugs (by increasing uric acid production with tumour breakdown), and alcohol.

<u>Allopurinol</u> prevents gout by reducing uric acid production through xanthine oxidase inhibition. It should not be started or stopped in acute gout, where sudden fluctuations in uric acid levels can worsen attacks. <u>Calcium channel blockers</u> (e.g. amlodipine), <u>ACE inhibitors</u> (e.g. ramipril) and <u>statins</u> (e.g. simvastatin) do not cause or worsen gout.

33. C. Folinic acid. Methotrexate inhibits the enzyme dihydrofolate reductase, which converts dietary folic acid to tetrahydrofolate (FH4). FH4 is required for DNA and protein synthesis. Folinic acid is readily converted to FH4 (without the need for dihydrofolate reductase) and is therefore useful in methotrexate toxicity. Folic acid cannot be used as in the absence of dihydrofolate reductase activity, it cannot be converted to FH4 and is therefore not metabolically useful.

Activated charcoal is only useful where poisons have been recently ingested (e.g. within 1 hour). Toxicity in this case has occurred over weeks. Haemodialysis is not useful in removing methotrexate from the circulation, although may be necessary when managing the associated renal failure. Granulocyte colony stimulating factor (G-CSF) has been used in the treatment of neutropenia due to methotrexate toxicity, but is not routinely part of initial management.

Methotrexate toxicity may be very serious and its management is complex. Advice should be sought from a poisons centre.

34. B. Dalteparin 5000 units SC daily. All patients admitted to hospital should be assessed for the risk of developing venous thromboembolism (VTE). Pharmacological prophylaxis should be prescribed if there are any thrombotic risk factors, provided the patient is not at risk of bleeding. This patient's thrombotic risk factors include her age, history of deep venous thrombosis, and likely immobility during her acute illness. The usual choice is a low molecular weight heparin (LMWH) prescribed at a 'prophylactic dose', such as dalteparin 5000 units SC daily or enoxaparin 40 mg SC daily.

LMWH is preferred over unfractionated heparin (UFH) because its effect is more predictable. However, it is eliminated by the kidneys so is less appropriate in patients with renal impairment. In these cases, UFH may be used. Aspirin is usually employed to prevent *arterial* thromboembolism, for example after a stroke. Its role in the prophylaxis of venous thrombosis is limited. Warfarin is used in the treatment of *established* VTE to prevent clot extension and recurrence. In this context, it is often initially combined with a LMWH. However, it is not employed routinely in inpatients to prevent VTE.

35. A. Carbamazepine. Warfarin is metabolised by cytochrome P450 enzymes. Carbamazepine is an 'inducer' of certain cytochrome P450 enzymes; that is, it interacts with the regulatory regions of the genes to increase their transcription. The resulting increase in the amount of enzyme allows warfarin to be metabolised more rapidly. This means that less warfarin is available to inhibit clotting factor production, so its anticoagulant effect is diminished and the INR falls. This puts the patient at risk of thromboembolic complications.

Valproate is a cytochrome P450 *inhibitor,* so its effect would be to *increase* the INR. Gabapentin and pregabalin are notable among antiepileptic drugs in having few drug interactions. Diazepam is a benzodiazepine which is used to treat acute seizures, but not for chronic seizure prophylaxis. It does not interact with warfarin.

The term 'cytochrome P450' refers to a family of enzymes. At undergraduate level you would not be expected to know about the individual members of this family, so it is reasonable to consider them collectively. Moreover, there is some cross-talk between the family members. For example, carbamazepine is a major inducer of CYP3A4 (the cytochrome P450 enzyme that, in general, makes the greatest contribution to drug metabolism), but like most other CYP3A4 inducers, it also induces CYP2C9 (the most important contributor to warfarin metabolism).

36. E. Trimethoprim. First-line options for an uncomplicated urinary tract infection (UTI) include trimethoprim, nitrofurantoin, and amoxicillin (a broad-spectrum penicillin). Remember that when prescribing trimethoprim, you should make sure that the patient is not pregnant. Trimethoprim is potentially teratogenic in the first trimester. Nitrofurantoin should be avoided in the latter stages of pregnancy.

Cefotaxime, a third-generation cephalosporin, and gentamicin, an aminoglycoside, have to be given intravenously, so are not indicated for outpatient treatment of an uncomplicated UTI. However, cefaclor, an orally-active second-generation cephalosporin, can be used as second- or third-line oral treatment for UTI (i.e. where first-line antibiotics do not work), and is an option for UTIs occurring in pregnancy. Ciprofloxacin is a quinolone that can be used as second- or third-line oral treatment for UTI or for complicated urinary tract infections, but should not be used first-line, as bacteria can easily become resistant to it. Unless their use is essential, quinolones should be avoided in pregnancy and in children as they may cause arthropathy. Macrolides, such as clarithromycin, have little activity against the Gram-negative organisms that commonly cause UTI, such as *Escherichia coli*. They are not known to be harmful in pregnancy.

37. B. Benzylpenicillin and flucloxacillin. In the clinical setting, antibiotics are chosen based on a 'best guess' as to the likely causative organism and antibiotic sensitivities. When infection is severe, being wrong with this guess and prescribing inadequate antibiotic treatment can be life threatening, so combination antibiotics are often prescribed to cover all likely eventualities.

Skin and soft tissue infections are most commonly caused by *Staphylococcus aureus* and Group A Streptococci (e.g. *Streptococcus pyogenes*). These bacteria are usually sensitive to flucloxacillin (a penicillinase-resistant penicillin) and benzylpenicillin (a 'standard' penicillin), respectively. As such, this combination is appropriate for severe cellulitis.

Amoxicillin (a broad-spectrum penicillin) and clarithromycin (a macrolide) are used in severe pneumonia to cover typical and atypical organisms, respectively. Cefotaxime (a cephalosporin) and aciclovir (an antiviral drug) are used in suspected intracranial infection to cover bacterial meningitis and viral encephalitis, pending a diagnosis from lumbar puncture. Co-amoxiclav (amoxicillin with clavulanic acid) and metronidazole are used in intra-abdominal sepsis to cover Gram-negative aerobic and anaerobic gut organisms. Co-amoxiclav and gentamicin (an aminoglycoside) are used in complicated urinary tract infections to cover Gram-negative organisms.

38. C. Doxycycline. A wide spectrum of organisms can cause community-acquired pneumonia, including *Streptococcus pneumoniae* (Gram positive), *Haemophilus influenzae* (Gram negative) and 'atypical' organisms such as *Mycoplasma pneumoniae* and *Legionella pneumophila*. The 'best guess' antibiotic for pneumonia therefore should ideally have a broad spectrum of activity to cover all these possibilities. Doxycycline (a tetracycline) is suitable because it covers Gram-positive, Gram-negative and atypical organisms.

Flucloxacillin is incorrect because it is a penicillinase-resistant penicillin with a narrow spectrum of activity, principally focused against *Staphylococcus aureus*.

The quinolone antibiotics, including ciprofloxacin, are generally reserved for second- or third-line therapy to preserve their usefulness, as bacteria easily acquire resistance to them. Ciprofloxacin is mostly effective against Gram-negative organisms, including *Pseudomonas aeruginosa*. Moxifloxacin and levofloxacin have greater activity against Gram-positive organisms and are therefore preferred for pneumonia.

Ertapenem (a carbapenem) and cefotaxime (a cephalosporin) are broad-spectrum antibiotics which have to be given by injection. They are reserved for severe infections and those associated with resistant organisms, such as hospital-acquired pneumonia in people with underlying chronic lung disease.

39. A. Benzylpenicillin. Penicillinases are a type of β-lactamase enzyme produced by the majority of staphylococci. They inactivate penicillins (e.g. benzylpenicillin) by breaking their β-lactam ring.

Flucloxacillin, a penicillinase-resistant penicillin, is more likely to be active against penicillinase-producing staphylococci because it has an acyl side chain that protects its β-lactam ring. It is the antibiotic of choice for straightforward staphylococcal infections. Vancomycin does not contain a β-lactam ring so is naturally resistant to penicillinases. It is reserved for more severe Gram-positive infections or those resistant to penicillins (e.g. meticillin-resistant *Staphylococcus aureus* [MRSA]).

Both co-amoxiclav (a broad-spectrum penicillin comprised of amoxicillin and clavulanic acid) and Tazocin® (a broad-spectrum antipseudomonal penicillin comprised of piperacillin and tazobactam) contain β-lactamase inhibitors. This improves their activity against penicillinase-producing staphylococci and, more importantly, β-lactamase-producing Gram-negative organisms.

40. D. Gentamicin. Aminoglycosides (e.g. gentamicin) accumulate in cochlear and vestibular hair cells where they trigger apoptosis and cell death. This can cause deafness, tinnitus and vertigo. Macrolides (e.g. clarithromycin) can also cause tinnitus and hearing loss, but this is rare and usually associated with long-term therapy. Other drugs that cause ototoxicity include vancomycin and loop diuretics.

41. E. Doxycycline. Tetracyclines (e.g. doxycycline) bind to calcium in developing teeth and bone. This can cause discolouration and/or hypoplasia of tooth enamel and theoretically could affect the developing skeleton. They should not be prescribed for women who are pregnant or breastfeeding or to children who have not yet formed their secondary dentition (under 12 years of age). The other antibiotics can be used in children if clinically indicated.

42. B. QT-interval prolongation. The QT interval is the time between the beginning of the QRS complex and the end of the T-wave. It mostly reflects the time taken for the ventricles to repolarise. The QT interval is said to be prolonged if, after correction for heart rate (by dividing it by the square root of the RR interval), it exceeds 0.44 seconds in men or 0.46 seconds in women. This is associated with an increased risk of a life-threatening arrhythmia called torsade de pointes, a form of ventricular tachycardia.

There are several causes of a prolonged QT interval. Drug causes include antiarrhythmics (e.g. amiodarone), antipsychotics (e.g. haloperidol), macrolide antibiotics (e.g. clarithromycin), and quinine. Combining drugs with QT-prolonging effects can be dangerous (clarithromycin with quinine sulfate for this patient) and should be avoided. A useful database of drugs that prolong the QT interval is maintained by the University of Arizona Center for Education and Research on Therapeutics at www.qtdrugs.org (accessed 24/2/14).

This patient is not taking any drugs that increase the potassium concentration, and is not at risk of seizures. Had she been taking a statin, there would have been a risk that clarithromycin could precipitate myopathy.

43. B. Ferrous sulfate. Tetracyclines bind to divalent cations. They should therefore be separated by at least 2 hours from doses of calcium, antacids or iron (e.g. ferrous sulfate). The interaction reduces absorption of both drugs, although the risk of subtherapeutic antibiotic concentrations is generally the greatest concern.

44. A. Amoxicillin. Amoxicillin (a broad-spectrum penicillin) is formulated for intravenous administration and can be given safely as a slow bolus injection or intravenous infusion (providing the patient is not allergic to penicillin). Clarithromycin (a macrolide), gentamicin (an aminoglycoside) and vancomycin all require slow intravenous infusion rather than bolus injection to minimise toxicity. As bolus injections, clarithromycin can cause phlebitis and arrhythmias; gentamicin can cause ototoxicity; and vancomycin can cause anaphylactoid reactions. Doxycycline (a tetracycline) is only available for oral administration.

In practice, antibiotic choice will be determined principally by the diagnosis (and therefore likely organisms and their sensitivities) and the severity of infection. The fluid volume associated with its administration would be an additional but secondary consideration.

45. D. Metronidazole. People taking metronidazole who drink alcohol may experience an unpleasant reaction, including flushing, headache, nausea and vomiting. This reaction is thought to be due to inhibition of the enzyme acetaldehyde dehydrogenase, preventing clearance of the intermediate alcohol metabolite – acetaldehyde – from the body. Alcohol should be avoided during and for 48 hours after metronidazole treatment.

Chronic excessive alcohol consumption can reduce absorption of doxycycline (a tetracycline), but this is less likely and less severe than the interaction with metronidazole. The other antibiotics listed here do not interact with alcohol. Nevertheless, this might be a good opportunity to discuss 'safe' alcohol consumption (maximum of 21–28 units per week for a man).

46. E. Serum gentamicin concentration. Gentamicin, an <u>aminoglycoside</u>, is a potentially dangerous drug. Its dosing should be guided by measurement of the serum gentamicin concentration. There are several approaches to monitoring once daily gentamicin therapy and you should consult local policies. However, the most common method is to measure the 'trough' concentration; that is, the lowest concentration expected during the dosage interval. This is taken 18–24 hours after the last dose, and should be <1 mg/L to minimise the risk of toxicity.

The other tests are less time-critical and, generally, measurement so soon after the start of treatment is unlikely to be particularly informative. Audiometry may be used in prolonged aminoglycoside therapy to monitor its effects on hearing, since aminoglycosides are ototoxic. C-reactive protein is an inflammatory marker which can be used to monitor for resolution of infection. Impaired renal function is common in severe infections and influences gentamicin dosing regimens. It is assessed using the estimated glomerular filtration rate (GFR) and the serum creatinine concentration, from which estimated GFR is derived. Estimated GFR may be more informative than serum creatinine concentration, but it can be misleading when the renal function is unstable.

47. A. Acetylcysteine. <u>Acetylcysteine</u> is a specific antidote for <u>paracetamol</u> poisoning. It is highly effective if started within 8–10 hours of the overdose. The decision about whether to administer acetylcysteine is guided by the nature of the overdose and the serum paracetamol concentration. If it was a single overdose taken at a known time, you should measure the paracetamol concentration 4 or more hours after the time of ingestion then compare this to a paracetamol poisoning treatment graph found in the BNF. If the concentration is above the treatment line, acetylcysteine is indicated. If the overdose was staggered (that is, the time between the first and last doses was more than 1 hour) or its timing is uncertain, you cannot interpret the paracetamol concentration. You then need to make a decision based on the amount of paracetamol ingested. If this exceeds 75 mg/kg, treatment with acetylcysteine is likely to be necessary.

<u>Activated charcoal</u> is given in paracetamol poisoning only if the patient presents within 1 hour of the overdose. Cyclizine is an antiemetic (see <u>Antiemetics, histamine H$_1$-receptor antagonists</u>). It may be an appropriate symptomatic treatment for his nausea, but it is not as important as acetylcysteine at this stage. Omeprazole is a <u>proton pump inhibitor</u> which is not indicated in this case. <u>Naloxone</u> is a specific antidote for <u>opioid</u> toxicity; it is not indicated in this case.

48. D. Temporarily stop acetylcysteine and give chlorphenamine. When administered intravenously at high doses (such as in paracetamol poisoning), <u>acetylcysteine</u> can cause an anaphylactoid reaction. Like anaphylaxis, anaphylactoid reactions are mediated by histamine and involve symptoms such as urticaria, angioedema and bronchospasm. However, in contrast to anaphylaxis they do not involve IgE antibodies. This means that the reactions tend to build up more gradually, such that they can usually be identified and treated before they become too severe.

At this stage, the management would be to stop the acetylcysteine and administer an intravenous <u>antihistamine</u> (H$_1$-receptor antagonist), such as chlorphenamine. Once the reaction has subsided, it is usually safe to restart the infusion at a lower rate. <u>Adrenaline</u>, administered by intramuscular injection, is the key treatment for anaphylaxis, but it is not required for anaphylactoid reactions unless they are very severe or the diagnosis is in doubt. Ranitidine is an <u>H$_2$-receptor antagonist</u> used to suppress gastric acid production. It has little, if any, role in the treatment of anaphylactic and anaphylactoid reactions.

49. D. 1 L glucose 5% with potassium chloride 40 mmol over 8 h; 1 L glucose 5% with potassium chloride 40 mmol over 8 h; 500 mL sodium chloride 0.9% over 8 h. The patient described in this scenario requires intravenous fluid therapy to cover his normal daily fluid and electrolyte requirements (often referred to as 'maintenance requirements'). For stable adult patients these are, roughly:

Water 30 mL/kg/day
Sodium 1 mmol/kg/day
Potassium 1 mmol/kg/day

These can be met using a combination of <u>glucose</u> 5% (which effectively just provides water), <u>sodium chloride</u> 0.9% (which provides water and sodium), and <u>potassium</u> chloride (which is given as an 'additive' in the other fluids). There are numerous ways of arriving at the appropriate amounts, but option D is a reasonable one. This will provide 2.5 L/day of water, 77 mmol/day of sodium and 80 mmol/day of potassium.

The other options are less satisfactory: option A provides only 1 L of water and no potassium; option B provides too much sodium and no potassium; option C provides too much sodium; and option E does not provide any sodium at all.

Different approaches need to be taken if the patient has already built up a fluid deficit (i.e. they are dehydrated); if they have additional ongoing fluid losses (e.g. due to diarrhoea); or they have an electrolyte abnormality, oliguria or renal impairment.

50. D. Sodium chloride 0.9% 500 mL IV over 10 minutes. This patient is sick and requires urgent review by a senior clinician. While arranging this, it would be appropriate to start fluid resuscitation. Intravenous fluid solutions containing sodium at a concentration similar to that in extracellular fluid, such as <u>sodium chloride 0.9%</u> and <u>compound sodium lactate</u>, are retained in the extracellular compartment. This means that, after distribution, a reasonable proportion (about 20%) of the fluid remains in the circulation, making them a viable option for fluid resuscitation. Compound sodium lactate contains a small amount of potassium (5 mmol/L). In most cases this is insignificant. However, in a patient with hyperkalaemia or anuria, who cannot therefore excrete potassium, this makes it a less appropriate choice.

Glucose 5% is widely used for simple fluid replacement but is a poor choice for fluid resuscitation. This is because it distributes throughout total body water, leaving only about 7% in the circulation. Human albumin solution is a <u>colloid</u> which is preferentially retained in the plasma. However, there is little evidence that the use of a colloid rather than a crystalloid makes any difference to clinical outcomes, and they are considerably more expensive. Moreover, albumin is not usually stocked on general wards. The time required to source it from elsewhere in the hospital is likely to be prohibitive to use in this setting. Sterile water is not used in fluid therapy because it is hypotonic, so can cause osmolysis of cells. It is, however, used for reconstitution and dilution of drugs.

The volume of fluid required for an initial fluid challenge is usually in the range 200–500 mL, infused rapidly (e.g. over 10 minutes). In patients with adequate cardiac reserve, 500 mL of sodium chloride 0.9% or compound sodium lactate is reasonable. If a colloid is to be used, options include human albumin solution and synthetic colloids, such as a modified gelatin. The initial volume is usually lower than that used for crystalloids (e.g. 100–250 mL infused rapidly).

Index of drugs